Prevention's
3·2·1
weight loss plan

Eat Your Favorite
Foods to Cut Cravings,
Improve Energy,
and Lose Weight

JOY BAUER, MS, RD, CDN

RODALE

© 2007 by Joy Bauer

Prevention is a registered trademark of Rodale Inc.

Rodale books may be purchased for business or promotional use or for special sales. For information, please write to: Special Markets Department, 733 Third Avenue, New York, NY 10017

Printed in the United States of America

Rodale Inc. makes every effort to use acid-free ⊗, recycled paper ♻.

Book design by Carol Angstadt

Photographs by Mitch Mandel/Rodale Images

Library of Congress Cataloging-in-Publication Data

Bauer, Joy.
    Prevention's 3-2-1 weight loss plan : eat your favorite foods to cut cravings, improve energy, and lose weight / Joy Bauer.
        p.   cm.
    Includes bibliographical references and index.
    ISBN-13 978–1–59486–585–5   hardcover
    ISBN-10 1–59486–585–X   hardcover
    ISBN 10 1–59486–586–8   paperback
    ISBN 13 978–1–59486–586–2   paperback
    1. Reducing diets. 2. Weight loss. I. Prevention (Emmaus, Pa.) II. Title.
RM222.2.B38587 2007
613.2'5—dc22   2007031097

Distributed to the trade by Holtzbrinck Publishers

2 4 6 8 10 9 7 5 3 1   hardcover

2 4 6 8 10 9 7 5 3   paperback

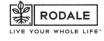

RODALE
LIVE YOUR WHOLE LIFE™

We inspire and enable people to improve their lives and the world around them

For more of our products visit **rodalestore.com** or call 800-848-4735

To my personal 3*2*1 plan:
my three kids, Jesse, Cole, and Ayden Jane;
my two parents, Ellen and Artie Schloss;
and my one and only husband, Ian

CONTENTS

Acknowledgments . . . vii

PART I: **THE 3-2-1 REVOLUTION**

CHAPTER 1 **Welcome to 3-2-1 Weight Loss** 3
It's realistic, effective, and oh, so delicious

CHAPTER 2 **3-2-1 Eating** 11
Consistent, regular meals boost metabolism and reduce hunger
and cravings

CHAPTER 3 **3-2-1 Fitness** 33
Burn fat, shrink your waistline, *and* sculpt muscle in one incredibly
effective workout

CHAPTER 4 **3-2-1 Motivation** 97
Daily strategies that ensure your success

CHAPTER 5 **Your Countdown to Success** 107
Weight loss goals that allow you to love your body—and love living
in your body

CHAPTER 6 **Pick Your Plan** 117
How to customize the plan for your body and your life

PART II: **PHASE 1**

CHAPTER 7 **About Phase 1** 127
What you need to know before you start

CHAPTER 8 **Phase 1** 141
What to do each day

CHAPTER 9 **Phase 1 Recipes** 177
14 quick and easy dishes that you'll love

PART III: PHASE 2

CHAPTER 10   **About Phase 2** 195
What you need to know before you start

CHAPTER 11   **Phase 2** 209
What to do each day

CHAPTER 12   **Phase 2 Recipes** 267
16 no-fuss recipes for the whole family

CHAPTER 13   **Plateau Pointers** 285
What to do if the scale stalls

PART IV: PHASE 3

CHAPTER 14   **Phase 3 Nutrition** 299
How to eat to keep off the weight

CHAPTER 15   **Phase 3 Fitness** 309
How to exercise to keep off the weight

3-2-1 Food Lists . . . 313

Selected Bibliography . . . 327

Index . . . 332

ACKNOWLEDGMENTS

Many people helped create this book and I'm eternally grateful.

Sincere thanks to Alisa Bowman. This book is a direct result of your hard work, dedication, and never-ending patience. You're a talented writer and I'm honored to work with you.

Tremendous thanks to my fabulous agent and friend, Jane Dystel. Special thanks to Miriam Goderich and the rest of the gang at Dystel and Goderich Literary Management.

Thanks to the entire crew at Rodale Publishing. Your enthusiasm and support are greatly appreciated. Special thanks to publisher and president, Liz Perl, executive editor, Nancy Hancock, and the rest of the editorial gang including Jenna Alifante, Courtney Conroy, Amy Super, Lisa Considine, Nancy N. Bailey, and Jane Sherman. Thanks to Carol Angstadt for a beautiful design and to Catherine Pawlowski for making it work out so nicely. Big thanks to fitness expert Michelle Stanton and to JoAnn Brader and the entire test kitchen staff. Sincere thanks to Liz Vacarella and the gang at *Prevention* magazine for believing in my work—it means a lot!

I'm eternally grateful to my friend and colleague, Leslie Dantchik. This book substantially benefited from your creative menu planning and hard work. Also, special thanks to Katherine Brookings.

Thank you to my attorney, Richard Heller—your input, direction, and legal advice is invaluable.

Many thanks to the 3-2-1 Weight Loss "test team": Anita Singh, Debbie McCullock, Earnestine Cole, Janice McGatlin, LeAnn Loche, Lori Wilson, Mary Idiens, Peggy Shackleton, and Tina Cundiff. Your enthusiasm (and weight loss!) made me smile. . . and your questions and input helped me work out the kinks.

Thanks to my wonderful family: Debra, Steve, Ben, Noah, Becca, Chloe, Harvey, and Jenny Beal; Ellen, Artie, Pam, Dan, Charlie, Cooper, Glenn, Elena and Otis Schloss. Carol, Vic, Harley, Jason, Mia, Jimmy and Lexi Bauer; Mary and Nat Malachowsky; Nancy Shapiro and Jon and Camrin Cohen; and of course, Lisi Eptein, Kael Goodman, Shannon Green, and Shamar.

I am forever grateful to my extraordinary parents, Ellen and Artie Schloss. You are my pillars of strength during every endeavor.

And last but certainly not least, thanks to my husband, Ian, and my three children, Jesse, Cole, and Ayden Jane. Your patience, understanding, and unbeatable support make every project possible.

PART I

The 3-2-1 Revolution

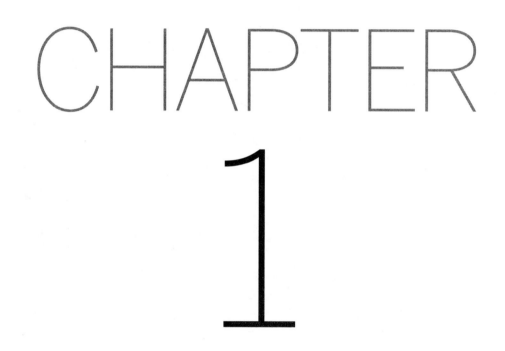

CHAPTER
1

WELCOME TO 3·2·1 WEIGHT LOSS

IT'S REALISTIC, EFFECTIVE, AND OH, SO DELICIOUS

Imagine a day—one not too far into the future—when you enjoy every delicious taste of breakfast, lunch, and dinner—without guilt or worry. On this day, you really and truly believe that while weight loss is certainly hard work, it's rewarding work. You, for once, are sure that you really can do this. You really can lose all the weight you want and continue to keep that weight off for the rest of your life.

On this new day, you complete your workout because you *want* to exercise. Rather than trying to distract yourself with television, music, or conversation, you find your exercise routine interesting and invigorating. You actually look forward to it.

At lunch, you go ahead and eat out with some friends. You don't worry about your eating plan because you know that you can follow it at any restaurant. You confidently order a meal that you know—without a doubt—will help you continue to lose weight.

At dinner, you finish what's on your plate, put your plate in the dishwasher without grabbing seconds, and leave the kitchen—without searching the freezer, cabinets, or refrigerator for something to satisfy your sweet or savory tooth.

During the evening, you pay bills, read, watch TV, or otherwise spend your time involved in something productive and worthwhile. You *don't* spend your time thinking about food.

At some point in the evening, you relax and savor a small serving of something incredibly delicious. Perhaps it's a few bites of chocolate, a glass of wine, or some chips with salsa. Rather than 3 bites turning into 20 bites and then 20 turning into the entire bag or container, you savor a few tastes and stop, knowing that you can taste this delicious food again tomorrow. You do not feel guilty. You do not lose control. You do not yearn for more. You do not head back to the kitchen. You don't even *think* about it. The noise that used to fill your head—*I want more, but I shouldn't have more, but I want more, but more will make me fat*—is gone. You go to bed feeling good about yourself. You wake up feeling refreshed and confident.

Oh, and your body; let's not forget that. On this day, you decide to try on that little black dress, that pair of jeans, whatever it is that you keep in the back of your closet *just in case you ever lose the weight*. On this day, you get out this article of clothing, pull it on, and feel the fabric easily slip over your more slender body. No pinching. No stuffing. No crinkling. No barely button-able buttons. It fits—and you look and feel beautiful.

This day can be yours. Really, it can. I've helped thousands of people have not one but many, many days just like it. For these clients, these wonderful days turn into weeks, the weeks turn into months, the months turn into years, and the years turn into the rest of their lives.

That's the promise of 3-2-1 Weight Loss.

It's effective. You'll lose up to 6 pounds the first week and up to 2 pounds each week afterward until you reach your goal. Participants who tried the weight loss plan before its publication lost between 3 and 6 pounds in Phase 1.

It's realistic. From Day 1, you have the option of eating out or in. From Day 1, you have the option of drinking moderate amounts of alcohol if you wish. From Day 1, you have the option of treating yourself to chocolate, popcorn, pudding, ice cream, chips, crackers, and much more—*every* day. From Day 1, you'll be able to prepare quick and easy meals that your family will love. From Day 1, you'll be able to modify the plan, making the meals you like and omitting the ones you don't. From Day 1, you'll be able to make the plan work for you, no matter what unique circumstances have prevented you from losing weight in the past.

It's invigorating. The fun exercise routine will keep both your brain and your body entertained.

It's delicious. You have a variety of mouthwatering menu options to choose from, plus the option of eating small portions of chocolate, chips, ice cream, pudding, pretzels, and other nondiet foods every single day.

It works. You will love every taste of it. I am confident that 3-2-1 is the last weight loss plan you will ever need.

WHAT IS 3-2-1?

The 3-2-1 weight loss plan is a way of life. It combines effective eating, fitness, and thinking into one winning formula.

3-2-1 eating: You'll boost energy and reduce deprivation and cravings by having **3** meals, **2** snacks, and the opportunity for **1** delicious treat every day. This consistent, regular eating plan will boost your metabolism and stabilize your blood sugar levels, preventing sudden surges and dips that can cause fatigue, headaches, cravings, and extreme hunger.

3-2-1 fitness: You'll boost your metabolism, burn fat, and stay motivated by completing multiple exercise circuits that include **3** minutes of cardio, **2** minutes of strengthening movements, and **1** minute of abdominal work. All told, you'll complete five circuits of 6 minutes apiece. By combining strength training and cardio into one complete body-sculpting, heart-pounding workout, you'll *double* your results. Research completed at Montana State University shows that circuit strength-training programs like 3-2-1 burn nearly twice as many calories as weight routines that require you to do multiple sets of each exercise, resting between sets. In fact, this research found that circuit workouts like 3-2-1 allow you to strengthen and tone your muscles to the same degree as traditional weight workouts—but in half the time. The 3-2-1 routines last 30 minutes and incinerate roughly 250 calories.

3-2-1 motivation: This menu of positive behavior techniques is easy to remember. Some you do **3** times a day (each time you eat a meal), **2** times a day (just before or during lunch and dinner), or just **1** time a day or week. These strategies will help you to avoid every excuse you've ever used to cheat, backslide, or avoid exercise.

WHAT YOU CAN EXPECT

I've organized the 3-2-1 system into three phases. Phase 1 lasts one week and will gently introduce you to 3-2-1 exercise as you switch to 3-2-1 eating. You can expect to lose up to 6 pounds during this phase.

Phase 2 lasts until you've lost all the weight you want. The meal plan itself spans two weeks, but you'll find the advice you need to follow 3-2-1 until you reach your goal. During this phase, you can expect to lose up to 2 pounds each week.

Phase 3 serves as your maintenance phase. This phase of the plan will teach you how to maintain your positive habits so the weight that you lost during Phases 1 and 2 stays off for the rest of your life.

Lose up to 6 pounds during the very first week, with slower 1- to 2-pound losses every week after that! That's impressive, but it's not what sets 3-2-1 apart from other diets you may have tried. You can lose weight quickly in any number of ways—remember the grapefruit diet, the popcorn diet, and others that enable rapid weight loss?

The secret of the 3-2-1 winning formula does not lie in the pounds lost on the scale. Rather, it lies in something much more subtle but also much more powerful. Unlike other diets, 3-2-1 maximizes your enjoyment as you lose weight. Don't get me wrong. Losing weight requires effort. That's a fact; never lose sight of it. But 3-2-1 *minimizes* the effort and *maximizes* the satisfaction. It makes weight loss as painless as possible. You will find no other system like it.

How does 3-2-1 do all of this? With the following unique and powerful benefits.

Less hunger, more satisfaction from every bite. At its core, 3-2-1 eating encourages you to eat regularly spaced meals and snacks. Research shows that people who eat more frequent meals weigh less than people who eat less frequently. On this plan, you'll focus five out of six eating opportunities on healthy, fiber-rich, vitamin-packed foods. You'll eat the right balance of wholesome carbohydrates, lean protein, and healthful fat to slow digestion, stabilize blood sugar, improve immunity, and bolster your overall health. You'll improve your energy and mood, minimize hunger, speed metabolism, and reduce uncomfortable cravings.

The opportunity to eat your favorite foods every day. You will feel good about your ability to savor foods you love in the right portions to enable weight loss. Once a day, you can eat a controlled portion of whatever food or beverage you can't live without, whether it's chocolate, popcorn, alcohol, or snack chips. This daily indulgence reduces the feelings of deprivation common with other diets, helping to curb cravings and bingeing. Because you will always know that the opportunity to eat delicious food is just hours away, you will no longer feel the urge to hoard and eat huge quantities of your favorite treats at once.

A sane meal plan for people with insane lives. This plan is not only effective but also realistic. Each day, you will find detailed meal suggestions that are quick and easy to prepare and taste out of-this-world delicious. But you also will learn how to alter this meal plan as needed. Going out to eat? No need to abandon 3-2-1. Just consult the extensive list of restaurant meal suggestions and continue to lose weight while dining out at your favorite restaurants. Work late and don't have time to prepare dinner? Make one of the 3-2-1 emergency options that take just minutes to prepare. Or heat up that 3-2-1 approved dinner you put in your freezer for days just like this. Your kids eat only chicken (at least this week)? Then mix and match meals and recipes, making only the chicken dishes and omitting the fish dishes. From Day 1, you will find detailed advice for making this plan work for you, no matter what curveballs life throws at you each day.

Invigorating, interesting, motivating, effective exercise. Whether you are a current couch potato, a veteran exerciser, or someone who falls somewhere in between, you are going to love the 3-2-1 way of moving. The 3-2-1 exercise system allows you to trade in tedious, lengthy, and sometimes ineffective weight room sessions for a home-based workout with dumbbells. Gone are the boring rest breaks and set repetitions of traditional workouts. Instead you'll complete multiple, mentally stimulating 3-2-1 circuits. In three sessions of 30 minutes a week, you'll strengthen all of your major muscle groups, incinerate 600 or more calories, and firm your abs. Unlike traditional gym workouts, you will keep your heart rate up during your entire exercise routine—burning fat while you strengthen your major muscle areas. According to research at Montana State University, this allows you to double your results in the same amount of time.

A faster metabolism. Research shows that circuit workouts like the one recommended in 3-2-1 get you fitter faster than traditional workout regimens. You not only crank up your calorie burn during the toning segments, you also continue to burn more calories after the conclusion of your final circuit. According to research completed at the National Institute of Occupational Health in Oslo, Norway, workouts like 3-2-1 elevate your metabolism for up to 48 hours after your workout as your body replenishes energy stores and removes waste products. This enables you to burn up to an additional 150 calories postworkout.

A plan customized to your fitness level. There's nothing more frustrating than trying to learn an exercise routine that is above your level of ability—or even one that feels too easy for you. We all want that perfect plan, the one that challenges us to improve without overchallenging us with sore muscles, extreme fatigue, and major discomfort. With 3-2-1, you have that perfect plan! This program gives you detailed advice for modifying the 3-2-1 routines based on your ability. You'll learn how to match the right resistance and intensity for you.

A system for staying motivated. I wish all you needed was a great eating and exercise plan. But, if you've ever tried to lose weight before, you know that sticking with a meal plan and keeping the weight off require a certain amount of motivation and creativity. That's why I've devoted an entire chapter to 3-2-1 motivation and another chapter to common problems that can get in the way of weight loss.

In these chapters, you will find unique motivational strategies that have worked for the thousands of weight loss clients I've counseled over the years. These strategies will help ensure that you follow the exercise and eating plans without fail. Curious about some of these unique strategies? Here's a sneak peek.

- Brushing, flossing, and placing whitening strips on your teeth after meals (particularly dinner) to prevent yourself from indulging in second and third helpings

- Rating your hunger halfway through meals to increase your sense of satisfaction and prevent accidental overeating

- Drinking two glasses of water before lunch and dinner to put yourself in a positive mindset for the meal

- Using a food interference list to prevent binges caused by stress or negative emotions

- Polishing your nails to prevent eating when you're bored instead of hungry

- Placing nibbles (bites of your child's leftover mac and cheese, tastes of your spouse's restaurant entrée, handfuls of candy or snack foods available in the break room at work) into a brown bag instead of your mouth

A LITTLE ABOUT ME

I have been a registered dietitian for many years and have built one of the largest nutrition centers in the country. I've counseled thousands of people seeking to lose weight. They include high-profile businessmen, celebrities, models, and Olympic athletes, but they also include regular folks like you. I've helped people lose from 5 pounds up to and beyond 100 pounds. I've worked with people who had diagnosed eating disorders such as binge-eating syndrome and night-eating syndrome. I've worked with those whose excess weight stemmed from bad habits rather than psychological problems, like those who overate a little at a time and needed a sane way to put an end to the problem.

I've worked with housewives who gained weight by nibbling on their children's leftover macaroni and cheese and spaghetti. I've worked with waitresses who were tempted to eat every time they picked up an order in the restaurant kitchen. I've worked with businesswomen who struggled to rein in their eating at business lunches and dinners.

I've worked one-on-one with children and adults, with people who *needed* to lose weight to control diabetes or heart disease and those who *wanted* to lose weight for a special occasion.

In other words, I've worked with women and men of nearly every age, ethnicity, weight, and background. I've even worked with people who—at first—didn't *want* to change. These folks begrudgingly stepped into my office after an enormous amount of hen-pecking from a spouse, family doctor, or boss. You know what? After they tried a personally tailored version of 3-2-1 for one week, even these folks decided to stick with it and lose the weight.

I say all of this so you can understand that I've heard every excuse in the book about why you can't lose weight, follow an eating plan, or exercise. I don't think there is a single excuse that I have not heard and solved for a client in the past. In your hands, you hold a book that takes the real-life challenges of weight loss and meets them with a winning lifestyle system. It's sane. It's realistic. It's effective. It works. Try it. With 3-2-1, you can't go wrong.

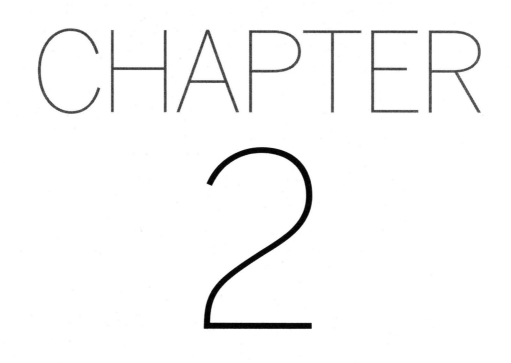

CHAPTER

2

3·2·1 EATING

CONSISTENT, REGULAR MEALS BOOST METABOLISM AND REDUCE HUNGER AND CRAVINGS

Welcome to 3-2-1 eating. I'm confident that this system of eating will revolutionize the way you think about weight loss. On this plan, you will eat the right foods at the right times in the right portions to reduce hunger and stabilize energy levels.

This plan will not only help you to shed fat in record time, but it's also good for your health, easy to maintain, and has already been proven successful by the many dieters I've counseled who have tried it. They tell me that this type of eating has helped them rein in cravings, overeating, emotional eating, and other barriers to successful weight loss.

To follow 3-2-1, you will abide by the following three golden rules of weight loss nutrition.

1. **Eat 3 meals, 2 snacks, and 1 (optional) delicious treat—every day.** Consistent, regular eating provides the cornerstone of 3-2-1 nutrition. Every day, you can have 3 meals, 2 snacks, and the opportunity for 1 delicious treat. You'll eat roughly every 4 to 5 hours. Research shows that people who eat frequent meals weigh less than people who eat less frequently.

2. **Make your 3 meals and 2 snacks 100 percent healthy (and delicious). Make your treat 100 percent delicious.** On this plan, you will fill each plate with the most healthful foods nature has to offer. The right balance of fiber-rich carbohydrates, lean protein, and healthful fat will satisfy your appetite, bolster your health, and promote a head-to-toe sense of well-being.

At the same time, each day you can indulge in a delicious treat of your choice at the time of day you most need it. Because you will always know that the opportunity to eat nondiet food is just a few hours away, you will better control the urge to eat huge quantities of your favorite treats at once. You may not always need your treats, but the opportunity to eat them is there for you every day just in case.

3. **Eat the right number of calories for your fitness level, age, and body size.** Some diets have popularized the notion that you can eat some foods in unlimited amounts as long as you keep a lid on your consumption of other foods. This is one of the biggest weight loss misconceptions ever advanced. No matter the unique makeup of a diet, calories matter. To successfully lose weight, you must eat fewer calories than your body burns. With 3-2-1, you will choose from one of three calorie-controlled plans, eating mouthwatering meals in the right portions to enable weight loss.

I've counseled many dieters who struggled to lose weight for years before seeking my guidance. In many of these clients, I've noticed a common theme. No matter what diets they had tried in the past, they typically hadn't combined all three golden rules into one successful eating plan. Some followed low-carbohydrate diets that provided lots of guidance about what foods to eat, but no guidance about portion sizes or meal timing. Others counted calories or points, but they did not pay attention to eating more nutritiously or regularly. Still others regimented their meal timing, going as far as setting an alarm to remind them to eat every few hours, yet they didn't always rein in calories.

Once these dieters switched to 3-2-1 eating and incorporated all three golden rules, the weight came off and stayed off without fail. Their stories are inspiring, and you'll read some of them in this chapter. It worked for them—and it will work for you!

RULE NUMBER 1:
3 MEALS, 2 SNACKS, 1 TREAT

As I mentioned earlier, eating the right food consistently throughout the day provides the cornerstone of 3-2-1 eating. Whether it's one of your 3 meals and 2 snacks or your 1 treat, you'll put food in your mouth roughly every 4 to 5 hours. This regular, consistent eating will balance blood sugar levels, keep your metabolism running smoothly, stabilize energy levels, and reduce between-meal hunger and cravings.

Although the research isn't in on precisely how frequently we need to eat to maintain our metabolism, energy, and self-control, I've found that most people must eat every 4 to 5 hours—and a few every 3 hours (these are people with a condition called *hypoglycemia,* or low blood sugar). Most dieters who do not have hypoglycemia can easily go 4 to 5 hours between meals without suffering the dramatic drops in blood sugar that lead to cravings, hunger, and fatigue. Spacing your meals this way allows you to make it from one meal to the next without feeling overpowering hunger, yet it does not require you to eat so frequently that you feel stuffed to the gills.

Let's take a closer look at this first golden rule of weight loss and how it will enable you to shed fat.

3-2-1 Preserves Your Metabolism

You want to do everything you can to preserve metabolism as you lose weight. As you lose weight, your metabolism will naturally slow down. It takes more calories to power a larger body than a smaller body. As you lose weight and become a smaller person, your metabolism adjusts to burn fewer calories. Also, as you lose weight, you will naturally lose some muscle tissue. Since each pound of muscle burns roughly 35 to 50 calories a day to maintain itself, losing any muscle mass can slow metabolism. Both of these weight loss effects contribute to the dreaded stalled weight loss that most dieters know as a *plateau.*

Regular eating habits will help to prevent that frustrating plateau by keeping your metabolism running smoothly. (Exercise will also help, but we'll get to that in Chapter 3.)

To understand how 3-2-1 helps preserve metabolism, we need to take a trip back in time. Human metabolism—the chemical processes involved in breaking down food and nutrients to produce the energy needed to build and maintain cell functions—has evolved over thousands of years. In the past 100 years, food has become plentiful, affordable, and available. Yet our metabolism still operates based on an archaic set of instructions left over from our distant hunting and gathering ancestors.

These ancestors could only survive—and pass on their genetic code—if their bodies were able to conserve calories when food was scarce. When these hunters and gatherers ran out of food, their bodies responded by slowing their metabolism. More specifically, the thyroid gland in the neck, which regulates metabolism, secreted a set of hormones that worked to slow calorie burning throughout the body.

Today, this mechanism still exists. As a result, when you go too long between meals or severely restrict your calories for days at a time, your thyroid puts the brakes on your metabolism. So you may be eating fewer calories, but you are also burning fewer calories.

Not only will regular meals preserve metabolism, they may even boost it through a process known as the *thermic effect of feeding.* When you eat, your body must burn calories to secrete digestive enzymes, break down food, and push it through your intestines. During digestion, some energy is also released as heat, which is why you may feel warm or even hot after eating a big meal. This thermic effect of feeding—the rate at which your body burns calories after a meal—accounts for roughly 10 percent of your total metabolic rate. Research shows that the thermic effect of feeding is higher when you eat regularly spaced meals.

In one of these studies, published in the *International Journal of Obesity Related Metabolic*

ROBIN: THE QUINTESSENTIAL NIGHT EATER

When Robin first came to see me, she was looking for help breaking an unhealthy eating cycle. She awoke each morning feeling bloated and full from snacking late into the previous night. She knew that breakfast was important, but she just couldn't stomach the idea of eating so early in the morning, especially after the huge number of calories she had consumed the night before. So she usually skipped it.

To make up for the previous night's indiscretions, Robin ate little to nothing for lunch. She might, for example, eat a small salad, a few raw vegetables, or a slice of toast. Not long into the afternoon, a headache (the result of low blood sugar) set in. She tried to work but instead fantasized about napping under her desk. To stay awake, she drank mug after mug of coffee, which contributed to feeling even more jittery and shaky. By midafternoon, she could think about only one thing—food—and her resolve to lose weight began to weaken.

Once Robin uncorked her urge to eat, she lost control. A candy bar from the vending machine led to cheese and crackers. Then a mocha latte. When she arrived home, she snacked on whatever was within reach as she prepared dinner. During dinner, she found she needed second helpings. After dinner, she broke out the pint of ice cream, with the cookies following close behind.

When I crunched the numbers, it was easy to see why Robin couldn't lose weight. She was eating as many as 2,000 calories after 7:00 p.m.! She was guilty of breaking the first cardinal rule of the 3-2-1 system: **She was not eating consistently throughout the day.**

When I suggested this new approach to Robin, she balked at first. She told me that she just could not eat breakfast, that she wasn't hungry at that time of day. In her mind,

Disorders, nine women changed their meal patterns multiple times during various two-week periods. They either ate six times a day or followed a haphazard schedule that included anywhere from three daily meals to as many as nine. The thermic effect of feeding 3 hours after a meal was lower when women ate erratically than when they ate regularly.

Finally, some research shows that regular, consistent meals and/or snacks eating five or six times a day—in conjunction with adequate protein intake (which you will learn about later in this chapter)—helps preserve muscle mass during weight loss. Because

Robin saw herself as a night owl and just assumed the night eating went along with that personality. She was also scared to death that the night eating would continue even after eating breakfast and lunch and therefore add even more calories and food volume to her day.

I asked Robin to try the 3-2-1 system for a week. If, after a week, she still felt as if she were choking down breakfast, she would be free to return to her old, weight-gaining ways. She agreed.

After a week, Robin returned to my office. She excitedly told me about the previous week. The first day had been tough. She didn't want to eat in the morning because she felt full and bloated, but she made herself. Later in the day, she noticed that she had more energy (and resolve). Her desire to crawl under her desk was gone. She was satisfied from her breakfast, and since she could look forward to a real lunch, she had no urge to visit the vending machine. During her dinner preparations, she resisted snacking. At dinner, she filled her plate just once. She saved a small treat for after dinner and was easily able to close down the kitchen by 7:00 p.m. The next morning, she woke up hungry—excited and entitled to eat breakfast. When she looked at her tummy, she realized that—for the first morning in a long, long time—she wasn't bloated. In fact, when she got dressed, she was able to tighten her belt one notch tighter!

"I'm amazed," she told me. "It took just one day for everything to change. I never would have believed it could be that easy." This simple change allowed Robin to eat more nutritiously and to eat smaller portions—changes that helped her to finally lose 15 pounds and to keep that weight off long term.

muscle tissue is a key factor in your overall metabolic rate, this effect is important. When you eat regularly spaced meals with appropriate amounts of daily protein, you help to ensure that most of the weight you lose comes from where you most want to lose it—your fat cells—and not from where you least want to lose it—your muscle tissue.

3-2-1 Weakens Your Cravings

In addition to signaling your thyroid to slow your metabolism, infrequent meals also can result in low blood sugar (known more technically as hypoglycemia). Low blood sugar triggers headaches, moodiness, dizziness, irritability, and fatigue.

Not only can such not-too-fun symptoms cause you to skip your 3-2-1 workout (because who in their right mind could exercise when they feel this tired?), but low blood sugar can also cause intense cravings that send you straight to the fridge. If you spend your mornings eating very little, you almost always wind up eating too much later in the day—usually at night. By 7:00 p.m. you feel ravenous, which leads to uncontrolled nighttime snacking.

When you eat regularly throughout the day, you provide your body with constant fuel, which reduces cravings and fatigue and helps you to find the willpower to eat the right foods in the right combinations at the right times. Your blood sugar levels remain in balance.

The 3-2-1 method reduces cravings for yet another reason. On this plan, each day you have the opportunity to have one controlled portion—about 150 calories—of your favorite food, whether it's chocolate or popcorn or wine or one of hundreds of other delicious foods or beverages typically banned on other diets. This treat reduces feelings of deprivation, setting 3-2-1 apart from other diets. With many diets, you go on them with the idea that you'll eventually go off them. Once you go "off" the diet, it's common to binge on whatever food you've resisted while dieting. In a study of 103 female students, published in the *International Journal of Eating Disorders*, students who were instructed to go a week without eating chocolate ended up eating *more* chocolate over the course of the week than students who were not told to restrict chocolate. In a similar study, participants who were told they would go on a diet the following day consumed more food in a test meal (the night before the so-called diet) than participants who were not told they would go on a diet.

The 3-2-1 system is different. You go on 3-2-1 to stay on it. On this plan, every day you will enjoy appropriate portions of the foods you love. You will never overindulge because you'll always know that you can eat more of the delicious foods tomorrow. Each day's treat allows you to feel satisfied and always gives you something to look forward to. It eliminates feelings of guilt that all too often lead to cheating, overeating, and binge eating. You will never again feel the need to punish yourself for "cheating" with skipped meals or think to yourself, "I blew it."

You may not believe that you can lose weight while still eating foods that you love—every day. Some of my clients didn't believe it at first either. When I suggested a daily treat to Linda, for example, she told me that having treats would make her fat. (She actually told me that she thought I was a "lunatic"!) Linda was an all-or-nothing thinker. To her, she was either on a diet—which meant she ate 100 percent perfectly healthy all the time—or she was off the diet, eating everything and anything. Linda did not see a middle ground. She told me she wanted me to design a strict, regimented plan that included no treats whatsoever.

Linda was convinced that eating treats would open a Pandora's box for her. She believed that the taste of delicious food would cause her to binge and abandon her diet. I could tell that she was firmly convinced, so I asked her to think about the possibility of adding a treat at a later date (treats that were *not* personal trigger foods for her), and then I let the issue go and designed the plan that she requested.

Linda started losing weight. After a couple of weeks, she told me she had cravings and would consider a limited list of treats. After talking with Linda more about her fears, I learned that she tended to lose control with certain types of foods—chocolate and chips. So I designed one treat list that included foods that she could eat—soft serve frozen yogurt purchased from a parlor (to keep the tempting pint out of her freezer), a miniature bag of light microwave popcorn, one serving of red licorice, 8 ounces of hot chocolate, and strawberries with whipped cream. I designed another list that included foods she should *never* eat—chocolate bars, cookies, snack chips, and any type of straight chocolate. These were foods Linda had binged on in the past and could become as problematic as she had feared.

The lists allowed Linda to maintain her sense of control over her diet but also allowed her the freedom to safely indulge. Amazingly, over time, she was able to increase the number of foods on her personal treat list, although a few specific foods remained off limits. She found that some days she needed her treats, and some days she didn't. Most important, she learned that she did indeed have control—something she hadn't felt in a long time. She was able to eat a single serving of her treat and stop.

You will be able to do the same. If you are like Linda and are unsure of your ability to stop eating a treat once you start, make a list of treats that aren't trigger foods to start. Give it some time. Eventually, you will find that you can add more and more fun foods to your list. You may even find, as some of my clients have, that you even gain control over those trigger foods. You may one day be able to eat a reasonable portion of *any* food without going overboard.

A Typical Day of 3-2-1 Eating

Everyone responds to 3-2-1 eating in a slightly different way. Most healthy people with normal blood sugar response can go 4 to 5 hours without eating and not experience low blood sugar. However, if you have been diagnosed with hypoglycemia, insulin resistance, prediabetes, or diabetes, speak with your personal physician. You may need to eat more closely spaced meals.

There's a big difference between following the 3-2-1 plan and grazing all day long. You will not be snacking mindlessly, reaching for whatever food you want when you feel like it. With 3-2-1, you will eat meals frequently enough to keep your metabolism humming along and to prevent cravings, but not so frequently that you overfeed your body and gain weight.

Each day of eating looks something like this, although the specific foods and portions will vary based on your lifestyle, metabolism, health, personal food preferences, and goals.

Breakfast: You may have heard that breakfast should be the largest meal of the day. You may even have heard the expression, "eat breakfast like a king, lunch like a prince, and dinner like a pauper." This advice is based on the theory that you can more easily burn off breakfast calories during the day—as you move around—than dinner calories, which you take to bed. In reality, there is no sacred calorie-burning clock. Although most people would probably function somewhat better if they could follow this meal-tapering philosophy, I've found that very few people can pull it off. Who wakes up feeling hungrier than they do at dinnertime? Most of us psychologically want dinner to be the biggest meal of the day. This is the time when we sit down with family, making the meal as much a ritual as a nutritional habit. For these reasons, the 3-2-1 breakfast includes just enough food to power you through your morning, but not so much food that you have to eat an unsatisfying dinner to meet your calorie goals.

Morning snack: The 3-2-1 meal plans include a morning snack to provide some holding power until lunch. If you eat breakfast late and lunch early, you may be able to skip this snack. If so, you have the option of eating this snack later in the day, whenever you most need it (as you prepare dinner or perhaps after dinner). On the other hand, if you wake early and eat lunch late, you absolutely need to eat your morning snack in the morning.

Lunch: The 3-2-1 meal plan includes a hearty lunch, a meal that contains lean protein to prevent a postlunch slump that often prompts the late-afternoon munchies. It also includes fiber-rich, high-quality carbohydrates to provide energy and slow digestion.

Afternoon snack: Eat this snack when you need it. I've found some people need theirs around 3:00 p.m. to prevent the midafternoon slump. Others do better if they save it until just before the commute home, as it prevents them from overeating at dinner.

Dinner: This largest meal of the day allows you to stay on the 3-2-1 plan and still enjoy a family dinner or even eat out. During Phase 1, 3-2-1 dinners contain a source of lean protein and lots of nonstarchy vegetables to fill you up and prevent late-night munchies. During Phase 2, most 3-2-1 dinners also include a high-quality, starchy carbohydrate food such as brown rice, quinoa, or baked potato.

Treat: Most of my clients like to have their treats either right after dinner as a dessert or a little later in the evening. Some even eat theirs right before bed (they save it for the last minute . . . in order to have something to look forward to). Have yours whenever it psychologically works best for you. Don't worry about the calories turning to fat as you sleep. This is a myth that has never been documented with research.

The 3-2-1 plan recommends specific portion-controlled treats. You don't *have* to eat your treats, but they are always there for you if you need them. After Phase 1, you will choose from a list of treats. *Always* stay away from your personal trigger foods, certainly during Phase 1 of the plan and until you feel in control. These trigger foods are the ones that you can't put down once you've started eating them. My clients' common trigger foods include ice cream in pint containers, large bags of chips, dry cereal, cookies, and peanut butter.

A Special Word for Night Eaters

Many of my overweight clients have a condition known as *night-eating syndrome*. These nighttime eaters generally consume more than half of their daily calories in the evening. When they wake up, they still feel full and bloated and as a result often skip breakfast. This fullness lasts for several hours after waking, and of course, they don't eat much during the day . . . and the cycle continues.

If all of this sounds intimately familiar, I have good news for you. You can break this cycle. I've seen it happen time and time again with hundreds of night eaters. Switching to 3-2-1 eating may at first be more challenging for you than for someone who doesn't snack excessively at night, but it's not impossible.

Your first strategy lies in eating breakfast. I know, I know. You aren't hungry in the morning. You're not a breakfast person. The thought of food first thing makes you sick. Yet, you must try to start the day with breakfast in order to break this nighttime eating cycle.

You might start with eating a small breakfast within 90 minutes of waking, perhaps half of what the 3-2-1 meal plan recommends. I know that eating anything in the morning is a big step for you. So, as long as you get nutritious food in your body in the morning, you are taking a big step in the right direction.

It's okay to skip the morning snack, but you absolutely must eat the prescribed lunch, afternoon snack, and dinner. I recommend that you eat your afternoon snack late in the afternoon, around 4:00 or 5:00 p.m. This will help to take the edge off, giving you more self-control at dinner.

Save your treat for close to bedtime. I've found that my clients who are night eaters tend to do better—at least in the beginning—if they have a treat to look forward to during the evening.

Many of my clients find that they begin to break the cycle almost instantly. Once they start fueling with the right food during the day (and know they have more food to look forward to every few hours—and the next morning), their urges to eat after dinner start to dissipate. Other clients, however, need to do more to break this cycle. If you find that after a week of eating breakfast, you still experience overpowering urges to eat at night, consult the tips for people with night-eating syndrome on page 290.

RULE NUMBER 2: 100 PERCENT HEALTHY MEALS AND SNACKS

As I've mentioned before, every day you will have the opportunity to indulge in delicious food that may contain very little in the way of nutrition. From cheese curls to cookies and everything in between, you can have it on the 3-2-1 plan as long as you follow the second rule of 3-2-1 eating. With the exception of your daily treat, the rest of your meals and snacks must be 100 percent nutritious. That means you will be eating real food—the stuff that grows in nature in the form of fruits, vegetables, whole grains, and legumes or comes from real animals in the form of lean meat or reduced-fat or fat-free dairy. You will also eat a balance of the three macronutrients—carbohydrates, protein, and fat. (*Macronutrient* simply means a nutrient that your body requires in large amounts, compared to *micronutrients,* which are vitamins and minerals that your body needs in smaller amounts.) The 3-2-1 plan is not a low-carbohydrate diet. It's also not a fat-free diet. Rather, it contains a healthful balance of these nutrients so that you can still enjoy the crunch and texture of your favorite healthful carbs, the delicious taste that can only come from fat, and the satisfaction that comes from protein. Yet, within each of these categories, you can make good and bad choices. So, to help you make the best choices, let's take a little refresher course in Nutrition 101, starting with carbs.

Carbohydrates: The Energizing Disease Busters

Carbohydrates include fruit, vegetables, starches (like bread and potatoes), and, of course, sugar. Despite what you may have heard or read in recent years, quality carbohydrates eaten in moderation will improve your health while making you look leaner and improving your energy levels. An essential nutrient, carbohydrates are the body's main source of both quick and sustained energy. Your body burns carbs during exercise, which is why you probably noticed you had little oomph in the exercise department if you've ever followed an extreme low-carb diet. Some parts of the body—red blood cells and some parts of the brain—can use *only* carbs for energy.

Carbohydrates also give you a big nutritional bang for your calorie buck. Of the three macronutrients, carbs are the only type that house fiber. Both types of fiber, insoluble and soluble, can help your weight loss efforts. *Insoluble fiber* provides volume to food without adding a lot of calories. Foods rich in insoluble fiber include high-fiber cereal, whole wheat bread, wheat bran, and fruits and vegetables. *Soluble fiber* helps stabilize your blood sugar levels, which in turn helps you better control your hunger and cravings. This type of fiber also slows the transit of food in your gut, creating a sensation of fullness for a longer period of time. Foods rich in soluble fiber include strawberries, apples, pears, oatmeal, chickpeas, and beans. Many studies have linked diets high in fiber with reduced body weight and body fat, yet less than half of adults consume the recommended 25 to 35 grams of fiber a day, and people who follow popular low-carbohydrate diets consume even less.

Some types of carbs also contain a lot of water. Fruits and veggies with high water content "built into the food" help to fill you up, so you'll eat less cumulatively throughout the day.

THE WHOLE PICTURE

Diets rich in whole grains have been shown in various studies to reduce the incidence of cancer, heart disease, diabetes, and obesity for the following reasons.

1. Whole grains are rich sources of fiber, resistant starch, and oligosaccharides that cannot be broken down and digested in the intestine. Although the research is mixed, it does appear that these nutrients may help to promote colon health.

2. Whole grains are rich sources of many vitamins, minerals, and plant nutrients that help reduce the incidence of heart disease and cancer.

3. Whole grains slow the absorption of carbohydrates into the bloodstream, helping to steady blood sugar levels.

In addition to fiber, carbs also house phytochemicals, important plant chemicals that enhance health and promote longevity. For these reasons, most 3-2-1 meals and snacks include high-quality carbohydrates.

All of this said, not all carbs are good for you or for your waistline. Some types of carbohydrates contain little to no nutritional value (think of high-sugar soft drinks), whereas other types of carbs are packed with fiber, vitamins, minerals, and phytonutrients (think spinach salad topped with chickpeas and various chopped veggies).

The 3-2-1 plan maximizes high-quality carbohydrates and minimizes low-quality carbs in your meals and snacks. On this plan, you'll eat carbs that closely resemble foods that grow in nature: fruits, vegetables, beans and other legumes, and whole grains.

In the whole grain category, you'll eat foods made from all three parts of the grain: the bran (the tough, fibrous outer layer), the germ (the nutrient-packed core of the grain), and the endosperm (the starchy middle layer). With the exception of your daily

PAM: THE JUNK FOOD JUNKIE

When Pam came to my office, she was under no illusions about what led to the extra roll of fat on her tummy. Pam ate regularly—a regular intake of junk. She started her day with pancakes and bacon, snacked on a buttered bagel in the morning, had a fast-food burger with fries for lunch, snacked on a candy bar in the afternoon, and finished the day with pizza. Instead of water, she drank soda, fruit juice, and other caloric beverages with meals.

Pam ate almost no vegetables, no whole grains, and no legumes. She was guilty of breaking the second cardinal rule of 3-2-1 eating. She was filling her plate with junk rather than nutritious foods that promote weight loss—and her waistline was responding by growing larger.

Pam wanted to change, but she didn't know how to turn things around. She didn't like how her body looked. She felt tired most of the time. Worse, her cholesterol levels were going up. It was her doctor who convinced her to come visit me. He told her if she didn't turn things around, she'd need to take medication.

Now, Pam loved her junk food, but as much as she loved the junk, she hated being fat and unhealthy. She was tired of the way junk food made her feel, but she felt overwhelmed by the prospect of change. When she plopped herself into the chair across treat, you will eat no refined grains, which do not contain the healthful layers and are composed entirely of endosperm. Refined grains may have finer texture, but they also have little to no fiber and very little natural nutrition. Examples include white flour and white rice, white bread, many crackers, and baked goods.

On the 3-2-1 plan, you will limit refined carbohydrates and simple sugars, like candy, jelly, and white rice, and anything made with white flour, like bread or pancakes (at least the ones that are not made from whole grain flour).

Refined carbs that are high in sugars are the most problematic, for both your health and waistline. Aside from providing empty calories, an influx of sugar into the bloodstream upsets the body's blood sugar balance, triggering the release of insulin, which the body uses to keep blood sugar at a constant and safe level. Prolonged elevated insulin levels can increase the risk for disease by causing inflammation within your body and by inhibiting key hormones that regulate the immune system. Insulin also promotes fat storage. All told,

from me, she actually said, "I don't expect to get anything out of this. I'm a lost cause."

As I tell most of my clients who doubt they can make a change, I told her to give me one week. I put Pam on a meal plan similar to the one you will find in this book. For her, I went a step further because I knew she wasn't used to cooking (beyond sticking a hot dog in the microwave). So I designed the meal plan to—at least in the beginning—include only healthful foods that required minimal kitchen preparation.

I also spent some time talking with Pam about her favorite foods, and I worked those foods into her meal plan as daily treats. Each day, Pam had that treat to look forward to. It helped her to stay on track.

Giving up soda and other flavored beverages was her toughest battle, so we took baby steps, allowing her to drink an unlimited number of diet beverages in the beginning.

After a week, Pam was back. She was a changed woman! She not only had more energy and a slimmer waistline, but she actually looked younger. She felt better than she had in years, and this positive energy motivated her to continue with 3-2-1 eating. "It's really worth it," she told me. "I feel so good, I don't miss the junk. In fact, I want to eat healthful foods now because I know how good they will make me feel!"

GIVING UP SOFT DRINKS

Many of my clients ask me whether they can use their daily soft drinks as their "treats." I highly discourage this for many reasons. First and foremost, you get only one treat a day. This delicious indulgence is sacred, one that should give you much more pleasure than what you would get from drinking a soda.

Soft drinks are a particularly rich source of sugar and high-fructose corn syrup (a type of sugar made from corn). One 20-ounce bottle of soda is the equivalent of pouring about 17 teaspoons of sugar straight into your body! What's more, those 250 empty calories are almost double the number of calories allotted for your daily treat.

By replacing soda with a nutritious beverage, you'll feel more energetic and satisfied, lighter on your feet, less bloated, and less moody. Better beverage alternatives include:

Water

Flavored water (with less than 20 calories per 8-ounce serving)

Plain and flavored seltzer

Fat-free and 1% reduced-fat milk

Soy milk

Green, black, and chamomile tea

Regular and decaf coffee

Skim latte, skim cappuccino, and skim café au lait

For optimal success, I encourage you to give up most sources of liquid calories. Pass on the soda, fruit drinks, smoothies (unless they're low calorie and accounted for), and coffee loaded with milk and sugar. Instead, drink lots of water and occasional diet beverages. For coffee, use fat-free or 1% milk and limit the sugar to one packet.

What Do I Do When the Only Carb Available Is Refined?

You can't eat perfectly all the time, and the 3-2-1 plan accounts for that. If you find yourself at a restaurant where the only rice they serve is white, you can still eat it. Just improve the rest of your meal with these two steps.

1. Round out your meal with digestion-slowing lean protein and a fiber-rich serving of vegetables.

2. Watch your portions and eat only ½ cup (about 3 heaping tablespoons) of the white rice.

when you have too many sugary sweets, you set the stage for rapid weight gain and elevated triglycerides, both of which have been linked to cardiovascular disease.

For those reasons, you should reserve sugary sweets for your daily treat. They're not 100 percent nutritious, so avoid them when planning your meals and snacks.

Protein: The Muscle Manager

Dietary protein comes from many sources, including animal meat, dairy products, eggs, and fish. It's also found in some carbohydrate-rich foods. For example, most whole grains contain some protein, as do many legumes.

Protein, made from combinations of 22 known amino acids, is an important building block of every cell in the body. It is an essential component of our DNA, hormones, and enzymes, and it makes up our bones, muscles, cartilage, skin, and blood.

All muscles in the body (including skeletal muscles, the heart muscle, and the smooth muscle that lines arteries and the digestive tract) need protein to repair themselves and do their jobs effectively. When you don't eat enough protein, your muscles do not have the amino acids they need to grow stronger and recover from exercise.

Dietary protein is important for weight loss for another reason. Protein slows digestion and the absorption of carbs into your bloodstream. This keeps blood sugar steady to prevent cravings and hunger between meals. In one recent study, researchers put 57 overweight participants on a diet that contained more protein and less fat. After 16 weeks on the diet, these participants reported experiencing fewer urges to eat after meals compared to other study participants who had remained on a diet than contained more fat and less protein.

Many studies show that high-protein diets actually cause participants to spontaneously eat less. In one of these studies, published in the *American Journal of Clinical Nutrition*, participants who doubled their protein intake reported feeling more satisfied after eating, and without even trying, they began eating roughly 450 fewer daily calories as a result.

Your digestive system also works harder to break down protein than it does to break down fat or carbohydrate. For this reason, protein tends to increase the thermic effect of feeding to a greater degree, which means you burn more calories after eating protein than you do after eating carbohydrates or fat.

You do not, however, have to go on a high-protein diet to experience this effect. Just do as 3-2-1 recommends and include lean protein at every meal. I need to stress the word *lean*. To lose weight successfully, you should avoid types of protein that are high in saturated fat (like bacon, pork or beef sausage, pepperoni, and prime rib and most other types of red meat).

In particular, avoid eating processed meats such as hot dogs, beef or pork sausages, and high-fat deli meats. Studies have linked these foods with an increased risk of type 2 diabetes, cardiovascular disease, and colon cancer.

The 3-2-1 plan optimizes the following healthful protein sources.

- **Fish:** Fish offers heart-healthy omega-3 fatty acids and, in general, less fat than many meats.

- **Poultry:** You can eliminate most of the saturated fat by removing the skin.

- **Eggs:** When you omit the yolk, you eliminate all of the fat and half of the calories.

- **Fat-free or reduced-fat dairy products:** Choose fat-free milk, fat-free yogurt, and reduced-fat or fat-free cheese.

- **Beans:** Beans contain more protein than any other vegetable source. Plus, they're loaded with fiber that helps you feel full for hours.

- **Nuts:** One ounce of almonds or other nuts gives you 6 grams of protein, which makes for a great snack. But be very careful with portions—nuts are very caloric.

- **Soy:** This plant protein is complete; it contains all of the amino acids that your body needs for good health.

Fats: The Feel-Full Factors

Different experts say different things about fat. Some weight loss diets allow unlimited fat, whereas others keep your consumption closer to zero. The 3-2-1 plan puts you somewhere between these two extremes.

Is It Possible to Eat Too Much Protein?

Unlimited protein can make you constipated (specifically when it displaces fiber-rich carbohydrates). Quality fiber is found in whole grains, fruits, and vegetables that are often in very short supply in high-protein diets. Fiber promotes bowel regularity, which reduces the risk of hemorrhoids, diverticulosis, and irritable bowel syndrome while lowering cholesterol and stabilizing blood sugar levels.

Controlling fat intake promotes weight loss because ounce for ounce and gram for gram, fat contains more calories than carbohydrates or protein. Carbs and protein supply 4 calories per gram, but fat supplies a whopping 9 calories per gram. In short, fat is fattening.

Yet, your body needs fat—especially certain types of fat—to run optimally.

You need fat to circulate and absorb the important "fat-soluble" vitamins: vitamins A, D, E, and K. Your body uses healthful mono- and polyunsaturated fats for energy, immunity, heart health, and mood and bowel regularity. Good fats also help your skin glow, give you shiny hair, and insulate and protect your vital organs.

In addition, fat slows digestion, helping you to make it from one meal to the next snack without feeling ravenous, and it makes food taste palatable. You will never be able to stick to your eating plan long term if your food doesn't taste good.

In short, depriving your body of fat is unhealthy and counterproductive for losing weight—yet, you must eat the right fats in the right quantities for success.

On the 3-2-1 plan, you will not add fat to your food, so don't think of fat as a food group. Rather, you will choose protein and carbohydrate foods that house healthful fats and minimize unhealthful fats. Most of your fats will come embedded in your food. You will eat omega-3 fatty acids in fish, monounsaturated fats in nuts and avocado, and polyunsaturated and monounsaturated fats in small amounts of salad dressing.

On the 3-2-1 plan, you will maximize the following fats.

• **Monounsaturated fats:** from avocados, olive oil, canola oil, and nuts

• **Polyunsaturated omega-3 fatty acids:** from fatty fish such as wild salmon (canned and fresh), mackerel (not king), trout, and sardines and from flaxseed, walnuts, and canola oil

At the same time, you will minimize saturated and trans fats. Eating too much of these unhealthful fats can raise blood cholesterol, which clogs arteries and increases your risk of heart disease. Saturated fats are found in marbled red meats, poultry skin, coconuts, coconut oil, palm kernel oil, and whole-milk products.

Trans fats, unlike unsaturated and saturated fats, do not exist in natural whole foods. They are created through a chemical process called *hydrogenation,* in which food manufacturers take unsaturated fats and turn them into trans fatty acids. This process is done to add to the shelf life of a product and change a food's texture. Yet studies have shown these chemically altered fats raise your risk of heart disease and arthritis. I recommend you eat as little trans fat as possible.

Food manufacturers know that consumers like you want convenient foods that are trans fat–free, so more and more snack foods now omit this type of fat. But not all of these "trans free" products are good for you. A product that claims to be trans fat–free is not necessarily low in saturated fat or sugar. It also may not be completely trans fat–free. The government requires that a product contain ½ gram of trans fat or less per serving to use the "trans free" claim on the label. If you eat multiple servings of a product that contains ½ gram of trans fat per serving, the grams of trans fat can easily add up.

RULE NUMBER 3: THE RIGHT NUMBER OF CALORIES FOR YOU

Portions matter. You can eat regular meals and snacks composed of the most healthful foods on the planet and still gain weight! I know because a client recently came to my office with this very issue. Her name is Lisa.

Lisa told me that she had been trying to lose 20 pounds for as long as she could remember. She had given up soft drinks, switched from refined grains to whole grains, and ate only lean protein. Her dietary choices revolved around vegetables, fruit, whole grains, beans and other legumes, and lean protein. She very rarely indulged in sweets. She never ate snack chips. She had banned junk from her home!

Lisa also exercised regularly and ate regular meals. On the surface, it seemed that she was doing everything right.

"I think there is something wrong with my metabolism," she told me. As it turned out, Lisa's metabolism was running normally, burning the usual number of calories for a fit woman in her early thirties. So, to get to the bottom of things, I asked Lisa to write down everything she ate for a few days. When I added up the calories she had recorded, I realized that Lisa was filling her plate with too much healthful food.

At breakfast, Lisa would eat whole grain cereal with milk and sliced banana along with a glass of orange juice. Yes, it's certainly a healthful meal, but Lisa generally poured herself not one but two servings of cereal, which alone added up to 240 calories. Her 8 ounces of orange juice came to 110 calories, the banana 110, and the milk 90. So, just at breakfast, Lisa was consuming 550 calories.

Then at lunch, she would eat a sandwich made of lean ham and low-fat cheese on a whole grain roll with mustard, lettuce, and tomato. Along with her sandwich, she'd have a salad topped with oil and vinegar. Again, the meal was healthy enough, but the calorie total was 750!

At dinner, Lisa would have a chicken stir-fry with brown rice. The meal itself was a great choice, but Lisa dished too much of it onto her plate, especially the rice. Dinner totaled 730 calories. Later in the evening, she ate a two-serving bag of popcorn, which added another 200 calories to her day.

The end result: Lisa was consuming more than 2,200 calories a day—for someone who needed to eat just 1,800 calories in order to lose weight. In the end, weight loss still comes down to a simple equation: Eat more calories than you burn, and you gain weight. Eat fewer calories than you burn, and you lose weight.

For Phases 1 and 2 of the plan, you don't need to worry about portions too much because you will follow a set meal plan designed for your optimal calorie intake. I urge you, however, to pay attention to the look of every meal before you consume it. It will give you an accurate picture of what each meal should look like when you start to maintain your weight in Phase 3.

It's important for you to know that there is no such thing as an all-you-can-eat weight loss plan. Successful weight loss requires that you follow all three of the 3-2-1 golden rules of nutrition. Omit any of these rules, and you slow or stall your results. Follow all of the rules, and you reduce between-meal hunger and cravings and lose all the weight you want.

3·2·1 TIP   **SPICE UP YOUR WEIGHT LOSS**   Research shows that you're often satisfied eating less food when the meal is spicy hot. Plus, you automatically eat slower and drink more water! If your taste buds can handle the heat, add chile peppers, hot sauce, and salsa to your meals.

3·2·1
SUCCESS STORY
Janice McGatlin

Age: 46

Accomplishment: Lost 9½ pounds, 1½ inches off her hips, and 1½ inches off her waist in seven weeks

Q: How did you gain the excess weight?

A: I am 46 years old with four children, one grandson, and one more on the way. I started 2006 30 pounds overweight, but it was nothing new. I had been carrying around 30 extra pounds for the last four years. It was time for a change.

Q: What weight loss plans had you tried in the past?

A: When I ran across the 3-2-1 plan, I had just lost some weight with the South Beach Diet. The 3-2-1 plan seemed less restrictive to me, however, and I wanted to incorporate some exercise. I am happy I was so selective.

Q: What changes have you noticed in your health?

A: I definitely have more energy, and I just feel healthier overall. I also look healthier—my skin is glowing (or so I am being told). Before I started the plan, I felt horrible. I would get up in the morning and be so stiff that I had to stretch just to get my body going.

Q: What changes have you noticed in your psychological health?

A: I now feel healthier and much better about myself than before I started the program. I feel more confident than I have in years. I feel really good about my health and just proud of myself overall.

Q: How did your hunger and food cravings on this plan compare with other programs you've tried?

A: I really like the flexibility of the diet plan, and I particularly like that it tells me what I *can* have rather than what I can't. For example, it offers a range of snack and treat options, and it tells me which foods to buy in the event that I don't feel like cooking the recipes. Also, my husband and I go to gourmet coffee shops like Starbucks often, and now I know which coffee drink options are acceptable for me.

Q: What did you think of the exercise?

A: I wanted to incorporate exercise into my diet plan, and the 3-2-1 program did it for me. I didn't have to think about what I needed to do—the workout guided me through it.

Q: Overall, what is your experience like with the 3-2-1 plan?

A: I really like this plan. It's different from others I've tried because it is flexible. It offers convenient recipes, meal plans, and substitutions. I particularly love having a dessert or treat and not feeling guilty about it because it's factored into the plan. The treats have been instrumental in my weight loss.

Also, I believe my success so far has been due to some of the other suggestions on the plan, such as journaling. I have journaled and kept a food log almost every day since I started—it was definitely an eye-opener for how many calories there really are in some foods!

Q: Would you recommend this program to a friend?

A: I would recommend this program to friends and family; in fact, I already have. My mother-in-law can't wait to start the program when the book is published. Thank you!

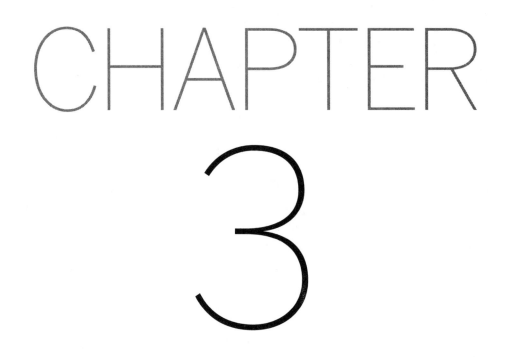

CHAPTER

3

3·2·1 **FITNESS**

BURN FAT, SHRINK YOUR WAISTLINE, *AND* SCULPT MUSCLE IN ONE INCREDIBLY EFFECTIVE WORKOUT

If you've ever asked a personal trainer to design a fitness plan for you, you may have received a one-routine-fits-all plan geared for guys. These exercise blueprints require you to:

1. Warm up for 5 minutes on a treadmill, exercise bike, stair climber, or other piece of equipment. You often skip it.

2. Stretch for roughly 10 minutes, targeting your major muscle groups (legs, back, chest, arms, and shoulders). If you do all of your stretches for the right amount of time, you congratulate yourself for your perseverance.

3. Hit the weight room, sharing the benches and dumbbells with big, sweaty guys who grunt loudly as they heft really big weights. You do a set of one exercise, rest for a minute, do another set of the same exercise, rest for another minute, do a third set, rest for a minute, and then move on to another exercise. Lift. Rest. Lift. Rest. You probably do one set and skip the rest.

4. Head back to an exercise machine for 20 to 30 more minutes of cardio. Usually, by this point in the routine, you're anxious to be done, but you coax yourself onto the treadmill because you know you get to don a set of headphones and watch *The Ellen DeGeneres Show* as you walk.

5. Cool down by slowing your pace and then stretching some more. At least, that's the plan. In reality, you're already in the locker room showering and changing.

The entire routine certainly includes all of the essential elements of exercise—fat-burning cardiovascular exercise (cardio), muscle-firming weight training, and muscle stretching—but it requires more than an hour of your time, and that doesn't even include the time it takes to drive to the gym, get changed, and then shower afterward. If you're like most people, it's a real challenge to fit the whole routine into your schedule.

The good news is that you can get all of the benefits of this approach—and more—by spending less time exercising. Even more enticing, you can reap all of these benefits at home, where you don't have to share your mat with *anyone* (short of perhaps your dog or young children). Now for the real kicker: You can trade in the boring lift-rest-lift-rest routine for a routine that keeps you mentally stimulated.

Enter 3-2-1 fitness. The 3-2-1 system allows you to trade typical weight room sessions for a home-based workout with dumbbells that includes 3 heart-pumping minutes of cardio followed by 2 minutes of strength moves and 1 minute of abdominal toning. You'll skip the boring rest breaks and set repetitions of traditional workouts and instead do multiple 3-2-1 circuits that will shape all of your major muscle groups. Unlike traditional gym workouts, this one will keep your heart rate up during your entire exercise routine—burning fat *while* you strengthen muscles. Now that's a workout!

BRING ON THE CARDIO

At the heart of 3-2-1 is a circuit training plan that gets you to do more cardio at a higher intensity. By combining strength training and cardio into one complete body-sculpting, heart-pounding workout, you'll crank up your routine. Here's how it works for each of the circuits.

3 minutes of cardio: During this segment, you'll jump rope and do other exercises that increase your breathing and heart rate so you burn more calories.

2 minutes of strengthening: Without taking a break, you'll pick up your dumbbells and zero in on one of your major muscle groups—arms, legs and shoulders, chest, buns, or back. Most of these strength-training moves require the use of your entire body and encourage you to tone more than one muscle area at a time. These combination exercises both strengthen your muscles and keep your heart rate elevated.

1 minute of abs: Again, without a break, you move right into any number of effective abdominal exercises to strengthen and tone your number 1 trouble spot. These abdominal movements also require effort, so again, your heart rate remains elevated.

All told, you'll complete five circuits of 6 minutes apiece. Although you're not doing official cardio during the entire 30 minutes of 3-2-1 circuits, your heart rate stays up the entire time. You not only crank up your calorie burn during the toning segments, you also continue to burn more calories after the conclusion of your final circuit.

By the end of the 30-minute routine, you will have burned more than 250 calories and sculpted all of your major muscle groups—all without leaving your house.

THE PROOF IS IN THE RESEARCH

Many studies show that this type of circuit workout beats out traditional exercise routines when it comes to weight loss. Consider:

- In a Montana State University study of 10 people, participants who did a 20-minute strength-training and cardio circuit workout burned nearly twice as many calories as participants who did a 20-minute weight routine in which they did three sets of each exercise and rested between sets.

- In a Japanese study of 35 healthy-weight adults, those who did a cardio/strength-training circuit lost 16 percent body fat, decreased bad LDL cholesterol by 19 points, and increased good HDL cholesterol by 11 points.

- For a Finnish study, researchers split 90 previously sedentary participants into three groups. One group made no changes. Another did a circuit with weight machines, moving quickly from one machine to another to keep their heart rates up to between 70 and 80 percent of their maximum rates. A third group did various forms of cardio (walking, jogging, cross country skiing, cycling) at the same heart rate intensity for the same amount of time. After 12 weeks of exercising three days a week, the circuit group had improved their cardiovascular fitness and strength to a greater degree than the cardio-only group.

This 3-2-1 exercise plan offers all of these benefits and more. By including an abdominal interval with every circuit, you will continually target the most common trouble spot. This is important. Unlike other muscles throughout your body, your abdominal muscles do not fatigue easily during exercise. You have just your body weight to use as resistance and a limited range of motion to apply that resistance. Often, when you try to work your abdomen with a series of movements back to back, other areas of your body (usually your neck, back, or hip flexors) fatigue first, causing you to use improper form and abandon the exercise before you've fully worked your abdomen.

By working your abs in short bursts repeatedly throughout the routine, you reduce the strain to your neck, hip flexors, and other small muscle areas and can more fully concentrate on proper form. This allows you to completely work your abdomen from every angle, maximizing your results. Specifically, you will:

- Flex your abdomen with crunch-like motions to strengthen the front of the tummy.

- Rotate your abdomen in twisting motions to target your waistline.

- Flex the sides of your abdomen (with side-bending movements) to further whittle your waistline.

By the end of your 3-2-1 routine, you will have moved your abdomen in all directions and worked it from every angle. You will feel the burn—and have a flatter, stronger tummy to show for it!

THE 3-2-1 ON THE THREE ESSENTIAL TYPES OF EXERCISE

During the 1980s, many women did just one type of exercise: aerobics. They donned leotards and leg warmers and danced, jumped, and stepped. In fact, I taught those classes all over Manhattan! Then came the 1990s, and women learned that they needed to do more than just burn calories. To prevent big age-related drops in metabolism, they also had to build muscle. In this muscle-building revolution, women were encouraged to check out and use the weight room—and many did. Some fitness plans even told women they could just lift weights and forget cardio (the newer, trendier term for *aerobics*) altogether.

Now we know better. As it turns out, you need a balance of both types of exercise—along with some stretching—for optimal results. Below, you'll learn more about the benefits of each.

Cardio: Plain and simple, cardio gets your heart rate up so you burn more calories. You burn between 80 and 100 calories for every 10 minutes of *vigorous* exercise. That comes to about 250 calories for 30 minutes and 500 calories for 60 minutes of high-intensity cardio. An hour of vigorous cardio can burn off an entire meal. Now that's motivation to move! Also, research shows that your metabolism may remain elevated for some time after your session, a physiological condition known as *afterburn*. The more intense your cardio (think 3-2-1 circuits!), the longer and more pronounced your afterburn.

FOR BEST RESULTS

The 3-2-1 fitness plan works somewhat like a state-of-the-art computer. It includes all of the state-of-the-art features but is only as effective as the person who sits and types at the keyboard. In other words, 3-2-1 provides everything you need to shape up and slim down, but you need to follow the plan correctly for the best results. To improve your metabolism, burn more calories, and stay motivated for your 3-2-1 sessions, you must tailor the workouts to your personal fitness level. In the following pages, you will find out how to do just that. Let's start with your training zone, the intensity at which you perform your workouts. As you'll learn, you must push yourself to achieve optimal results.

Weights: Each pound of muscle can burn up to 50 calories a day to maintain itself, making muscle an important determining factor in your overall metabolism. Yet, because of inactivity coupled with the natural aging process, most adults start to lose muscle mass, starting sometime after age 30. This muscle loss (called *sarcopenia*) accelerates as we age, particularly after menopause. Many physiologists estimate that a women in her 70s has lost at least 20 percent of the muscle mass that she had during her youth.

When you lift weights, you help to stall this loss of muscle, thus preserving the metabolism of your youth. The 3-2-1 circuits help to build this needed muscle strength, helping to boost your metabolism 24 hours a day.

Stretching: If you've ever attended a gentle yoga class, you may have noticed that the people who appeared to be the least fit had a much easier time getting their noses to touch their knees than the more heavily muscled of the bunch. This is no coincidence. Unbalanced training makes you less flexible over time if you do nothing to counteract it. Stretching helps to preserve your natural flexibility. In addition, stretching helps to prevent injuries and reduce muscle tightness. In the 3-2-1 plan, you will stretch during a cooldown at the conclusion of every workout.

Stay within Your Training Zone

The nature of the 3-2-1 routine will help to boost your heart rate somewhat automatically. That said, you should push yourself, resisting the urge to daydream as you go through the motions.

To do this, consider keeping track of your heart rate during your sessions, especially during the first few weeks. If you have a heart rate monitor, this task will be automatic and easy. Just place the monitoring strap underneath the bottom edge of your sports bra, then periodically check the watch on your wrist as you work out to see how often your heart is beating per minute.

If you don't have a heart rate monitor, you can check your heart rate manually. Just place a finger or two against the carotid artery in your neck to find your pulse. You'll find it between your collarbone and jaw line. Count the beats for 6 seconds and then add a zero to whatever number of beats you counted to determine the number of beats per minute.

THE 3-2-1 ON YOUR TRAINING ZONE

It's one thing to know what heart rate you want to achieve during your workout but another to actually hit it. Read below to find answers to common training zone problems.

"I can't get my heart rate high enough!" Push yourself harder during your cardio segments. You might even scrap the suggested movements (perhaps your level of fitness is higher than the routine allows for) and instead do high-energy, heart-pumping cardio in the form of jumping rope. Also, you can speed up your movements (but keep them controlled to avoid injury) during the 2-minute toning segments to increase your burn, but *always* slow down for the 1 minute of abdominal work. Proper form at a slower speed is mandatory for ab moves, as you will more effectively target your muscles.

"My heart rate is too high!" If you are out of shape, you're probably overdoing it. Consider taking a break or doing the cardio segment at a lower intensity, especially if you find that you get so fatigued that you can't finish the entire routine. On the other hand, if you are highly fit, your target heart rate may actually be higher than the 226-minus-your-age calculation. As long as you feel energized at the end of the routine, continue to exercise at this intensity.

You want the beats per minute to stay within a specific training zone of 60 to 75 percent of your maximum heart rate. This training intensity will maximize not only the number of calories you burn during your workout but also the number of calories you burn after your session (the so-called afterburn). To determine your training zone, subtract your age from 226. (*Note:* You may have seen formulas that subtract your age from 220. These formulas are designed for men, not for women.) Then multiply your answer by 0.7. This is the maximum number of times you want your heart to beat per minute during your 3-2-1 routines.

After a couple of weeks of keeping track of your heart rate, you'll have a better idea of what your training zone should feel like. After that, go by feel. If you hit a plateau, however, start monitoring your heart rate again. You may have begun to slack off.

Listen to Your Body— And Alter the Routine as Needed

No matter your fitness level, I recommend you start with the Phase 1 routine and see how it feels. This routine includes the beginner and low-impact versions of various exercises. For example, in the Phase 1 routine, you'll do pushups on your knees. In Phase 2, the routine takes things up a notch, suggesting pushups with your legs fully extended.

If after your first time through, the 3-2-1 routine feels too easy, then you just passed your advanced placement test and can move directly to the Phase 2 routine. Think of it as starting college at the sophomore level. On the other hand, if Phase 1 feels challenging, stick with this routine for at least a week—and possibly longer. It's perfectly fine to stick with the Phase 1 fitness routine even if you have moved on to the Phase 2 meal plan.

Your goal is to eventually do both the Phase 1 and the Phase 2 routines without taking breaks between segments. Depending on your level of fitness, however, you may need to rest every once in a while to catch your breath. This is fine. Do what works for you, pushing yourself just a little bit harder during each exercise session. To continually motivate yourself, consider wearing a stopwatch to time your rest breaks. Each time you do the routine, use the feedback from your watch to shorten your rest breaks. For example, let's say during your first week with the 3-2-1 routine, you must rest for a minute between circuits. During Week 2, try to cut your rest break to just 50 seconds. Then, in Week 3, to 40 seconds, and so on.

Put In the Right Amount of Time for You

You will use the following weekly schedule. This schedule is designed to work a beginner up from no fitness to higher fitness.

Phase 1: Do the 3-2-1 workout three days a week, taking a day off between sessions.

For example, do the workout each Monday, Wednesday, and Friday. If you are already exercising three days a week, you have a choice. You can either do the 3-2-1 workouts *instead of* your current exercise sessions, or you can do them *in addition* to your current sessions. Listen to your body (not to mention your life commitments) and do what you will most be able to sustain long term.

Phase 2: Increase to three or four days a week, taking a day off between sessions. For example, exercise every other day (Sunday, Tuesday, Thursday, Saturday, and then the following Monday, Wednesday, Friday).

Phase 3: At least one of your four sessions a week, do the routine twice, for a total of 60 minutes. This will burn roughly 500 calories per session. Also, add some power walking to your week, fitting it in during your days off from 3-2-1.

Wield the Right Weight for You

The 3-2-1 plan requires minimal equipment: You need only a set of dumbbells. For your comfort, you might also want to invest in an exercise mat.

For the dumbbells, use the information below as a basic guide, designed for beginners who need to build more strength. As a general rule of thumb, you should feel fatigued after working each muscle area. Your goal is to work until muscle failure—the sensation that you couldn't possibly lift the weight again. If your muscle does not feel warm and you never feel the burn, the weight is too light. If you have trouble executing a movement with proper technique, cannot do the full range of motion for an exercise, or feel a sharp pain in any of your joints, the weight is too heavy.

If you already have a basic idea of the amount of weight you can handle, go with that amount.

Phase 1: Use a set of 3-pound weights and a set of 5-pound weights. Use the heavier weights to exercise larger muscle groups such as your chest, legs and upper back, and biceps. Use the lighter weights to strengthen the smaller, weaker muscles in your triceps and shoulders.

Phase 2: Once those weights begin to feel too light, you are ready to move up. Start using 5-pound weights for your smaller muscle areas and purchase heavier 8-pound weights for your chest and other large muscle groups.

Phase 3: Depending on how the routine feels, consider moving up in weight again, using 8- and 12-pound sets of weights.

Avoid These Common Mistakes

The 3-2-1 routines are fast and effective, allowing you to get the same results as from traditional programs in half the time. That said, on very busy days, you may find yourself tempted to shorten the routine by skipping the warmup or cooldown or by doing only the circuits that target your trouble spots. Resist the temptation!

For best results, you really do need to do the entire routine.

The importance of your warmup: These gentler cardio exercises in the beginning of the routine will slowly get your heart rate up to your training zone. Unlike the engines of high-end sports cars, the human heart just isn't designed to go from 60 to 140 within seconds. Your warmup also does exactly that: It raises the temperature of your muscles, making them more pliable. This prevents straining your muscles as you execute complicated movements. It also reduces postexercise muscle soreness. More important, your warmup eases your mind into your workout. You may find at the beginning of your workout that you just don't feel like exercising. On these days, tell yourself that you will just complete the warmup and that if you still feel dreadful, you'll take the day off. Generally, at the end of the warmup, you'll be ready for more. You won't want to quit.

The importance of doing all of your circuits: The 3-2-1 routines work all of the major muscle groups in your body equally. This helps to prevent muscle imbalances that can lead to soreness and injuries. Do all of them, not just those for the body areas you wish to tone.

The importance of the cooldown: Your cooldown includes your stretches. On the 3-2-1 plan, you stretch your muscles at the end of the routine, when they are warm and least prone to injury. Stretching them at the beginning or at other times of the day when they are cold can lead to tissue tears.

THE 3-2-1 ROUTINES

So now that you know about the effectiveness of the 3-2-1 routines, you are ready to get acquainted with the exercises you'll be doing over the course of the next several weeks. In the following pages, you will find two complete routines to use during Phase 1 and Phase 2 of the overall 3-2-1 plan. (When you get to Phase 3, you will find advice in Chapter 15 for designing your own unique 3-2-1 circuits.) The routines outlined in the following pages share the same warmup and cooldown. They also share many exercises, making them easy to remember. The Phase 2 routine simply takes movements from the Phase 1 routine and cranks them up a notch to help increase your fitness and calorie burn.

The 3-2-1 Warmup

Do the following warmup before both the Phase 1 and Phase 2 routines. It will gently ease you into your routine, reducing your risk of muscle pulls or other injuries. As an alternative to the following suggested movements, you can simply march in place, walk on a treadmill, or use some other piece of exercise equipment for 3 to 5 minutes.

MARCH

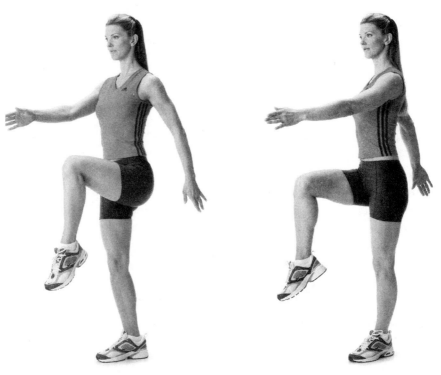

Stand with your feet under your hips and your hands at your sides. Start marching, lifting your left knee toward your chest, lowering it, and then lifting your right knee. Lift your knees as high as possible. As you march, pump your arms back and forth. March for 1 minute.

WIDE ROLLING SQUAT

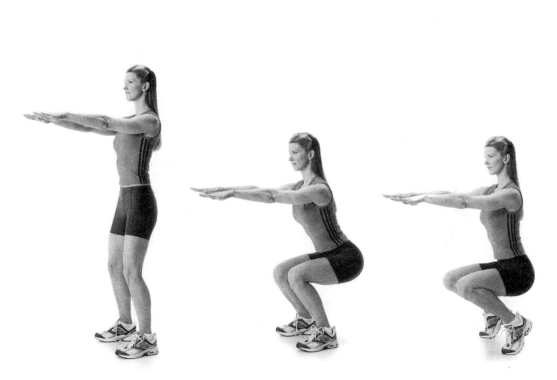

With your feet slightly wider than hip distance apart, bend your knees and squat down, lifting your arms out in front at shoulder level as you do so.

Hold your squat as you lift your heels and rise onto your toes. Lower your heels, straighten your legs, and repeat. Continue this movement for 1 minute.

TORSO TWIST

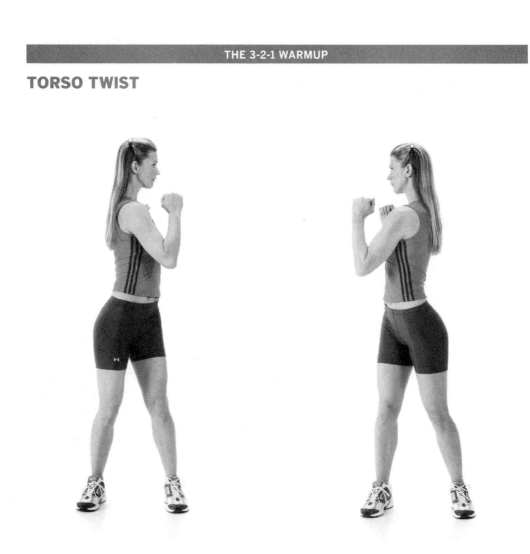

With your feet slightly wider than hip distance apart, bend your elbows, bringing your hands to shoulder height. Bend your knees slightly and twist your torso to the left and then to the right, keeping your spine long as you twist. Twist fairly quickly, taking just a second to twist in each direction. Continue for 1 minute.

REACH AND PULL

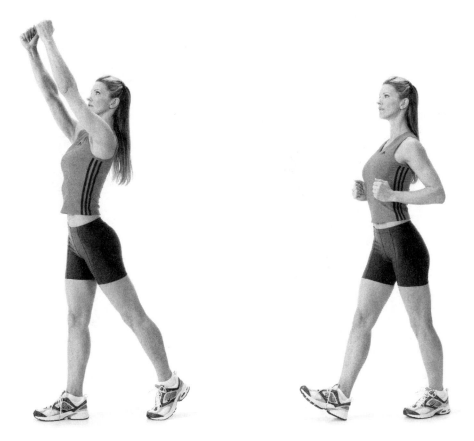

Stand with your feet in a scissors position, with your right foot about 2$\frac{1}{2}$' in front of your left. Extend your arms overhead as you shift your body weight forward, allowing your left heel to rise.

Lower your arms (as if you were pulling a cable down to your hips) as you shift your body weight back onto your left leg, allowing your right forefoot to rise off the floor and bending your left knee. Repeat for 30 seconds in this position and then switch so your left leg is in front.

BEND AND ROUND

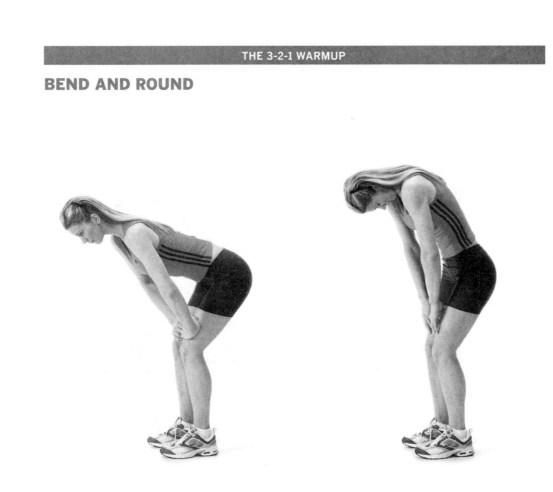

With your feet slightly wider than hip distance apart and your knees slightly bent, place your palms on your thighs and bend forward from the hips with a flat back. Once your torso is parallel with the floor, round your back. Then exhale as you roll up one vertebra at a time, lifting your head last. Do this three times.

The 3-2-1 Arms Circuit

Your arms circuit will shape your biceps and triceps, the pair of muscles that form your upper arms. Your biceps is the brawny muscle in the front of your arm that so many of us like to flex in a display of our fitness. The triceps is at the back of the upper arm. This common trouble spot tends to get flabby with age. This 3-2-1 circuit will shape and firm your arms so you will feel confident in sleeveless shirts and spaghetti strap dresses.

3-MINUTE CARDIO

PHASE 1: MARCH

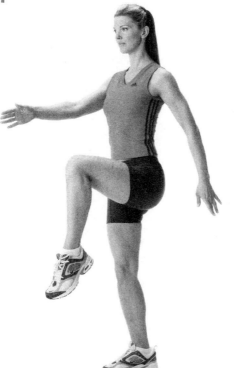

Stand with your feet under your hips and your hands at your sides. Start marching, lifting your left knee toward your chest, lowering it, and then lifting your right knee. Lift your knees as high as possible. As you march, pump your arms back and forth. March for 1 minute.

PHASE 2: **JOG**

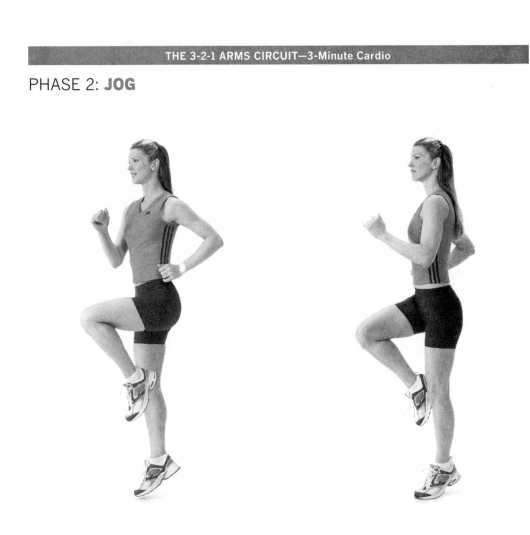

Starting with your feet under your hips, jog, pumping your arms and lifting your knees as high as possible. Jog for 1 minute.

PHASE 1: **JUMP ROPE**

Pick up an imaginary jump rope and, with your hands at hip level, begin to "swing" it around your body. Move through the following footwork sequence for a total of 2 minutes as you twirl your rope, making sure to keep these movements low impact by not jumping with your standing leg. In Phase 2, you'll add a hop to boost heart rate.

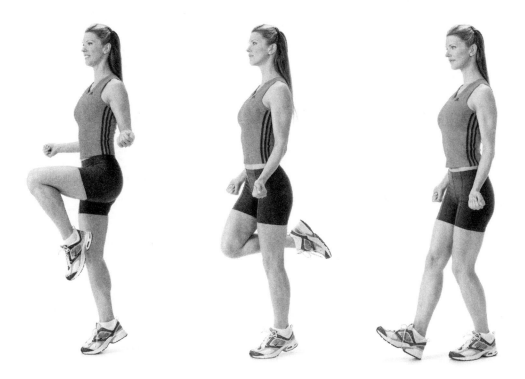

HIGH KNEES: Bend your elbows and bring your hands toward shoulder level as you jump with high knees, lifting one knee toward your chest, then the other. Try to keep the move low impact for now, just hopping slightly each time you raise a knee but not allowing your standing forefoot to launch itself into the air. For a lower-impact version, keep your toes on the ground and lift your heels alternately, switching from right heel to left heel.

JOG: As you twirl the rope, jog with your feet, bringing one foot at a time toward your buttocks.

STEP: As you twirl the rope, step forward with your right leg, lifting your forefoot and tapping your heel to the floor. Bring your right leg back to meet your left, then step forward with your left foot.

PHASE 2: **JUMP ROPE**

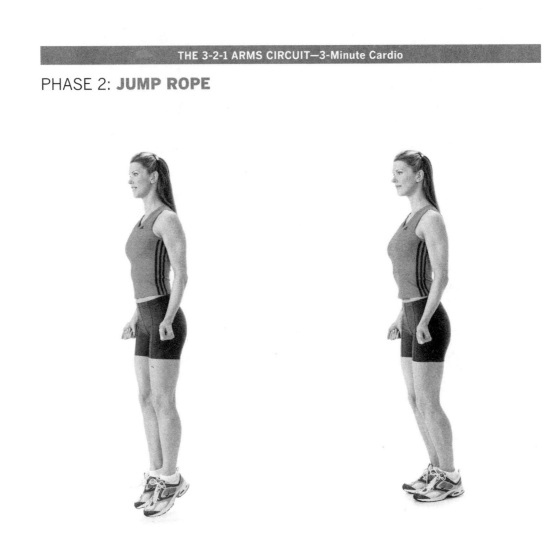

Pick up your imaginary jump rope and, with your hands at hip level, begin to "swing" it around your body. Then, for 1 minute, jump with both feet off the floor as the rope swings around. To keep your brain entertained, you may alternate these standard jumps with any of the legwork options described in Phase 1. Just take things up a level by adding a true jump to all of those moves and getting air time for those feet!

PHASE 1: **STEP TOUCH**

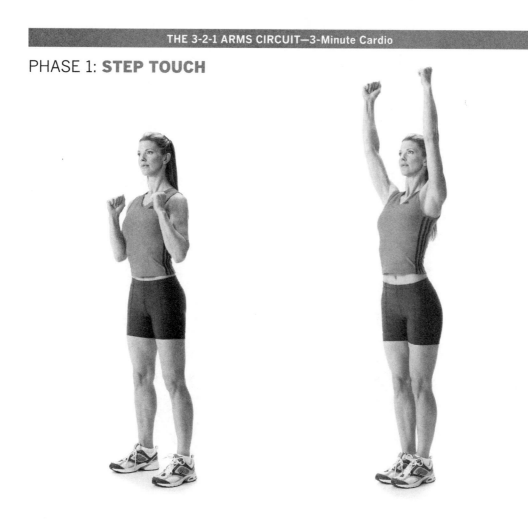

Starting with your feet slightly wider than hip distance apart and your hands at shoulder level with your elbows bent, step your right foot toward your left, raising your arms overhead as you do so.

Step your right foot back out, bringing your feet into a wide stance and lowering your arms as you do so. Then step your left foot toward your right, repeating on that side. Continue to step right and left for 1 minute.

PHASE 2: **STEP HOP**

Similar to the step touch you completed during Phase 1, these step hops will really get your heart racing.

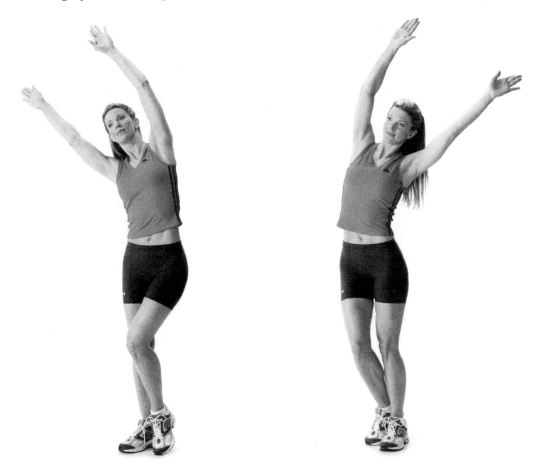

Starting with your feet slightly wider than hip distance apart and your hands at shoulder level with your elbows bent, hop your left foot toward your right, moving your arms overhead from left to right as you do so.

Then, without returning to the wide stance, hop one foot at a time to the right, moving your arms from right to left as you do so. Continue hopping left to right for 1 minute.

2-MINUTE STRENGTHENING

PHASE 1: BICEPS CURL

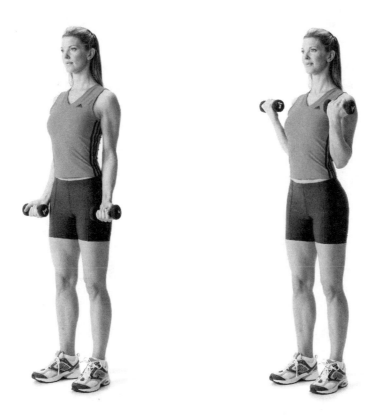

Stand with your feet under your hips, with your knees soft but not bent. Grasp a dumbbell in each hand with your arms extended by your sides and your hands near your hips, palms facing forward.

Keeping your elbows close to your sides, bend your elbows and curl your hands toward your shoulders, then lower. Repeat for 1 minute.

PHASE 2: **BALANCING BICEPS CURL**

You learned how to do standard biceps curls in Phase 1. Now you will continue with this exercise, but you'll increase the challenge by standing on one foot. Doing so will force you to firm your abs and core as you curl, allowing you to accomplish two goals at once!

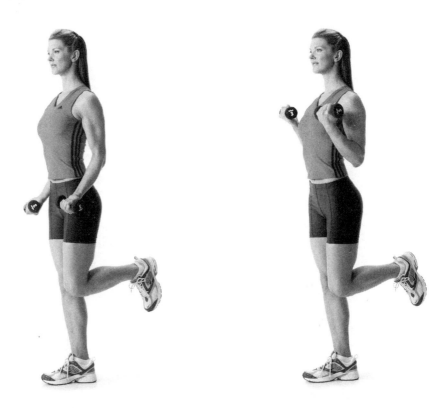

Stand with your feet under your hips. Grasp a dumbbell in each hand, with your arms extended by your sides and your hands near your hips. Shift your body weight over your right foot. Bend your left knee and lift your left foot off the floor. Then, keeping your elbows glued to your sides, bend your elbows and curl your hands toward your shoulders, then lower. Repeat for 1 minute.

PHASE 1: **TRICEPS DIP**

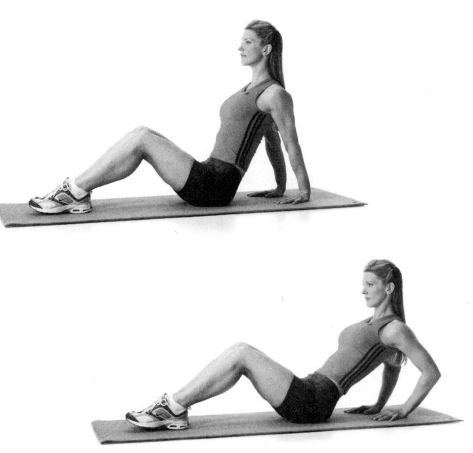

Sit on the floor with your knees bent and your feet flat on the floor. Place your palms on the floor 6" to 12" behind your buttocks with your fingers pointing in. Sit tall, with firm abdominals and a long spine.

Bend your elbows as you lean back, feeling the work in the backs of your arms (the part that jiggles when you wave), then rise. Repeat for 1 minute.

PHASE 2: **TRICEPS DIP II**

This exercise is similar to the triceps dip you did during Phase 1. You will now lift your hips off the mat to increase the challenge of this move.

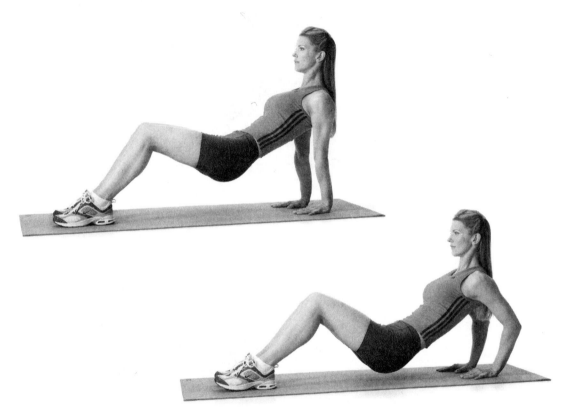

Sit on the floor with your knees bent and your feet flat on the floor. Place your palms on the floor 6" to 12" behind your buttocks. Sit tall, with firm abdominals and a long spine. Press into your palms as you lift your buttocks about 6" off the floor. Bend your elbows as you lower your buttocks toward the floor (without allowing them to touch). Then rise as you straighten your arms. Repeat for 1 minute.

1-MINUTE ABS

PHASES 1 AND 2: DANDASANA TWIST

Don't let the simplicity of this twist on a standard yoga posture fool you. This twist will do wonders for your waistline!

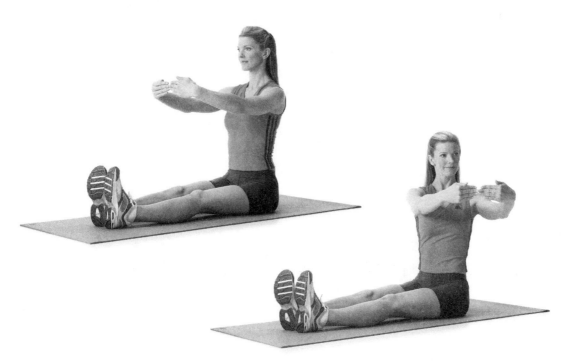

FOR BOTH PHASES: Sit with your legs extended, your abdominals firm, and your spine long. Squeeze your feet together and flex them. Extend your arms in front at shoulder level, with your fingertips touching.

Keeping your spine long, your tummy pulled into your spine, and your arms directly in front of your chest, twist to the left, holding for a count of 3-2-1 as you exhale in three quick breaths. As you exhale, focus on using your tummy muscles to blow out the air. Then return to center and repeat on the right. Continue alternating left and right for 1 minute.

The 3-2-1 Legs and Shoulders Circuit

The following heart-pumping, efficient circuit will sculpt and firm your legs and shoulders simultaneously. These combination movements require you to strengthen your arms as you strengthen your legs with movements that will test your coordination and boost your heart rate. The lunges, in particular, are one of the most effective movements for firming the thighs—another common trouble spot for many women. The plié squats will also help to firm the thighs, targeting the typically flabby inner thighs as well as the backs of your thighs just under your buttocks—the roll of flab that tends to hang out of the bottom of your bathing suit! The shoulder raises will sculpt the fronts, tops, and backs of your shoulders, creating a sexy shape that will make you regret ever having to cover them up!

3-MINUTE CARDIO

PHASES 1 and 2: HEEL TOUCH

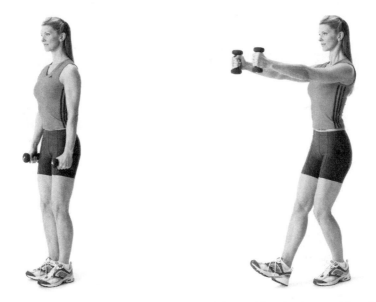

FOR PHASE 1: Stand with your feet under your hips and hands at your sides. Grasp a light dumbbell in each hand. Step your right foot forward, flexing your foot and tapping your heel to the floor. At the same time, lift your arms in front to shoulder level. Step your feet back together and then repeat by stepping your left foot forward. Continue alternating right and left for 1 minute.

FOR PHASE 2: Do the exercise as described in Phase 1, but to increase the intensity, add a hop as you switch feet.

PHASE 1: JACKS

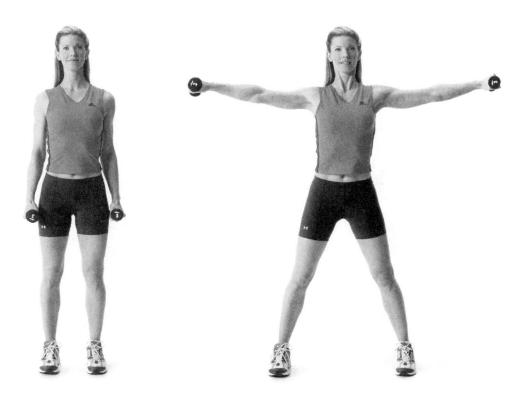

Grasp a light dumbbell in each hand. Place your hands at your sides and your feet under your hips. Bend your knees slightly and step to the right with your right foot, raising your arms to the sides at shoulder level as you do so. Bend your knees, then lower your arms and step your right foot back to the left before repeating with your left foot. Use the slight bending and straightening of your knees to add a "hop" to your jack, but don't allow your forefoot to get airtime. Continue alternating right and left for 1 minute.

PHASE 2: **JACKS**

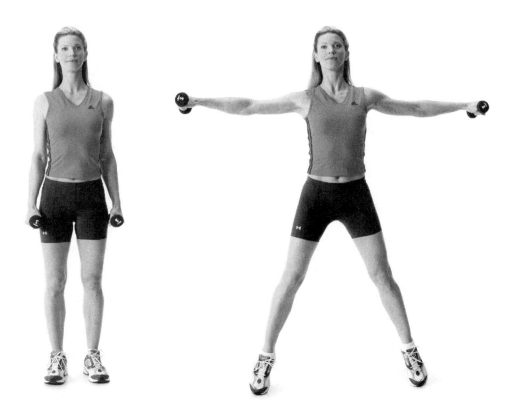

Grasp a light dumbbell in each hand. Place your hands at your sides and your feet under your hips. Jump your feet apart into a wide angle as you raise your arms to the sides at shoulder level. Lower your arms as you jump your feet back together. Continue jumping out and in for 1 minute.

PHASES 1 and 2: **HAMSTRING CURL**

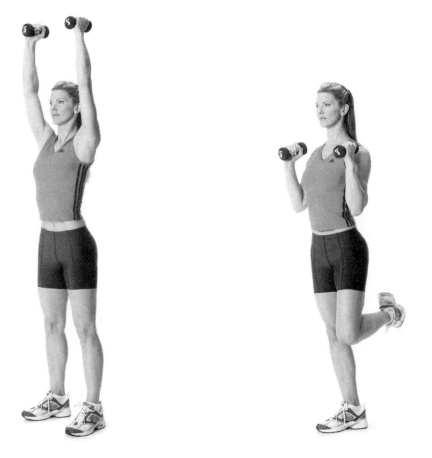

FOR PHASE 1: Grasp a light dumbbell in each hand. Stand with your feet slightly wider than hip distance apart and extend your arms overhead. Shift your body weight over your right foot as you lift your left foot, attempting to kick your buttocks with your left heel. As you do so, lower your arms. Then raise your arms and repeat with the other foot, alternating sides for 1 minute.

FOR PHASE 2: For this move, you'll continue with the same exercise described in Phase 1. If you'd like to really rev up your heart rate, consider adding a hop to each leg curl.

2-MINUTE STRENGTHENING

PHASES 1 and 2: **LUNGE WITH SHOULDER PRESS**

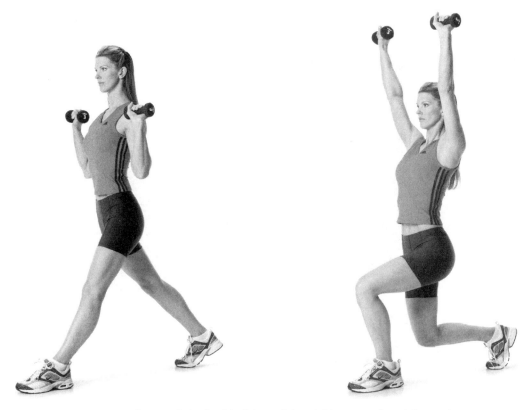

FOR PHASE 1: Grasp a light dumbbell in each hand. Move your legs into a scissors position, with your left foot about 2½' in front of your right. Bend your elbows, placing your hands at shoulder level with palms facing forward. Lift your back heel, moving onto the ball of that foot.

Bend both knees, lowering your back knee toward the floor and keeping your front knee over your ankle. As you lower, extend your arms overhead. Rise and repeat for 30 seconds before switching sides.

FOR PHASE 2: Continue with the lunges from Phase 1. If you'd like to increase the challenge, do a knee lift with your front leg when you come to a standing position.

PHASES 1 and 2: PLIÉ SQUAT WITH SHOULDER RAISE

This exercise gives you a lot of bang for your buck. It will help you to lift those buns, firm your inner thighs, and shape your shoulders—all in one move.

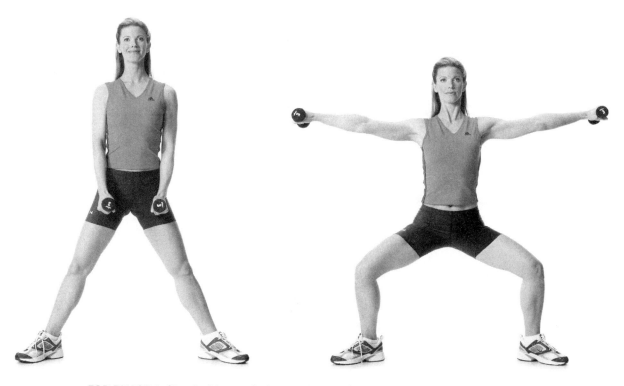

FOR PHASE 1: Stand with your feet spaced about 2' apart. Grasp a light dumbbell in each hand and turn your toes out and heels in. Place your hands just in front of your hips.

Exhale as you bend your knees, tuck your tailbone, squeeze through your buttocks, and squat down. As you do so, raise your arms to the sides at shoulder level. Rise as you lower your arms. Repeat for 1 minute.

FOR PHASE 2: Execute the move as described in Phase 1, but during the final 15 seconds, sink down into the plié squat and hold. Place your hands at your hips for support. Lift and lower your heels for 15 seconds, then rise and move on to the abdominal segment of the circuit.

1-MINUTE ABS

PHASES 1 AND 2: **ROLL BACK**

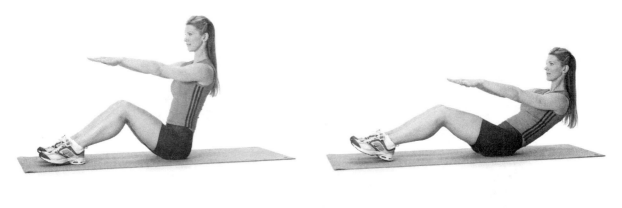

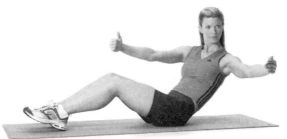

FOR PHASE 1: Sit on a mat with your knees bent and your feet flat. Keep your knees and feet directly in front of your hip bones; don't allow your knees to splay outward. Lift your arms in front to chest level. Beginners can hold onto the backs of their thighs for extra support.

Curl your spine, rolling back from your tailbone to your lower back. Concentrate on scooping out your abs as you roll back. Rise to the starting position. Repeat for 30 seconds.

FOR PHASE 2: To firm the sides of your abdomen, you will continue to roll back as you twist to one side. From the starting position, curl your back, scoop out your abs, and roll back as you rotate your torso to the left and open your arms to the sides. Rise as you return to center, then repeat to the right. Continue alternating left and right for 30 seconds.

The 3-2-1 Chest Circuit

By now, you should really be starting to feel the power of this workout! Your heart is beating, your muscles are singing—and you've still got a few more circuits to go! This circuit will tone your chest, an often-neglected muscle area for many women. The pushups and flies in the strength segment will build up your pectoral muscles, creating the illusion of cleavage for you gals who are not naturally endowed. It also can help to lift and add some shape to your breasts. The bicycles suggested for the abdominal portion are among the most effective abdominal exercises, proven by research. Do them slowly, and you'll see the results.

3-MINUTE CARDIO

PHASES 1 AND 2: FRONT JAB

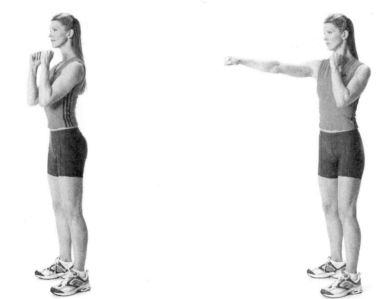

FOR BOTH PHASES: Stand with your feet slightly wider than hip distance apart. Bend your elbows and bring your fists close to your face (to protect your face from your opponent!). Bend your knees, squatting down slightly.

Rise, and as you extend your legs, shift your body weight to the left as you throw a jab with your right hand, as if you were trying to punch someone directly in front of you. Do not lock your elbow as you punch. Bring your arm back as you bend your knees slightly, then repeat with a left jab. Continue alternating right and left for 1 minute.

PHASES 1 AND 2: **FRONT HOOK**

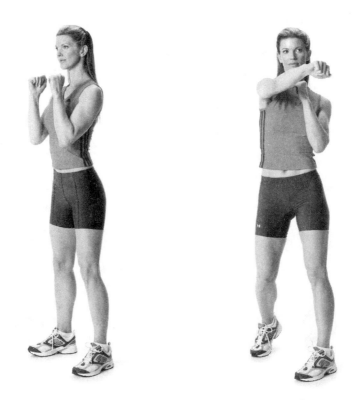

FOR BOTH PHASES: Stand with your feet slightly wider than hip distance apart. Bend your elbows and bring your fists close to your face (to protect your face from your opponent!). Bend your knees, squatting down slightly.

Rise, and as you extend your legs, shift your body weight to the left as you throw a hook with your right hand, as if you were trying to punch someone in the side of the head. As you throw the hook, your fist should come up and around in an arc. Rotate your torso as you punch. Bring your arm back as you bend your knees slightly, then repeat with a left hook. Continue alternating right and left for 1 minute.

PHASES 1 and 2: **KNEE STRIKE**

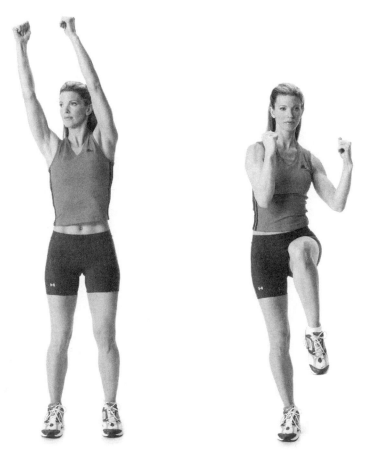

FOR PHASE 1: Stand with your feet slightly wider than hip distance apart. Lift your arms overhead and to the right.

As if you were grabbing something and smashing it into your knee, thrust your arms downward as you lift your left knee. Lower and repeat once before switching sides. Continue to do two strikes on each side—alternating sides—for 1 minute.

FOR PHASE 2: Do the move as described in Phase 1, but to increase intensity, add a hop to the move as you lift your knee.

2-MINUTE STRENGTHENING

PHASE 1: KNEE PUSHUP

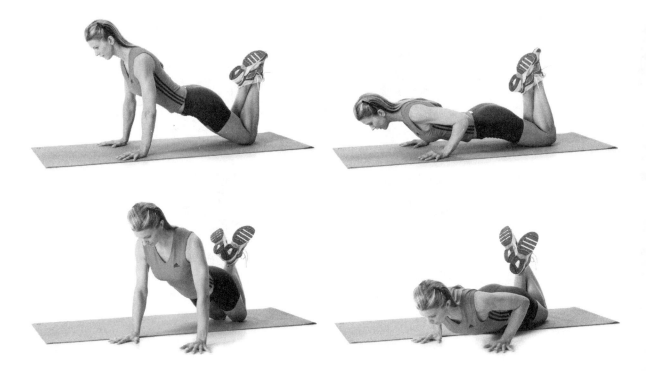

Kneel with your hands on the floor, slightly wider than shoulder distance apart. Lift your lower legs off the floor and cross them at the ankles. Lean forward, forming a straight upward diagonal line from your knees to your head.

Bend your elbows as you bring your chest to within an inch of the floor.

Rise and walk both hands to the left, bringing your torso off-center. Bend your elbows and lower your chest to within an inch of the floor. Rise, then walk your hands back to center. Do a pushup at center and then walk your hands to the right. Do a pushup, then walk your hands back to center. Continue alternating center-left-center-right-center for 1 minute.

PHASE 2: **ADVANCED PUSHUP**

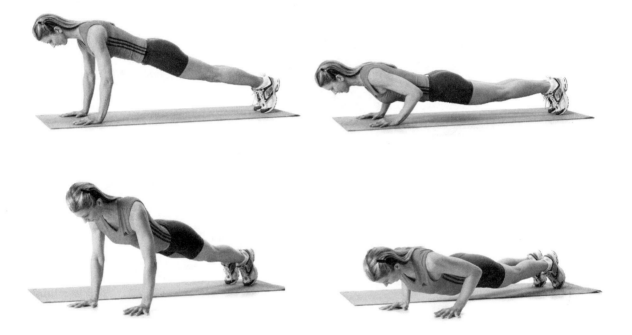

Bring your body into a plank position, with your legs extended and supported on your toes and your hands on the floor, slightly wider than shoulder distance apart. Reach out through your heels and the top of your head, creating a straight diagonal line from your heels to your head.

Bend your elbows as you bring your chest to within an inch of the floor.

Rise and walk both hands to the left, bringing your torso off-center. Bend your elbows and lower your chest to within an inch of the floor. Rise, then walk your hands back to center. Do a pushup at center and then walk your hands to the right. Do a pushup, then walk your hands back to center. Continue alternating center-left-center-right-center for 1 minute.

PHASE 1: **CHEST FLY**

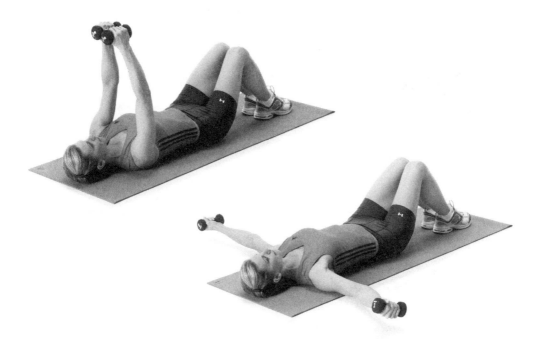

Lie with your back on a mat, with your knees bent and your feet flat on the mat. Grasp a light dumbbell in each hand. Extend your arms so your hands are above your chest with your elbows slightly bent.

Open your arms to the sides, moving slowly to a count of 3-2-1. Squeeze through your chest as you bring your hands back together, as if you were hugging someone tightly, moving slowly for a count of 3-2-1. Repeat for 1 minute.

PHASE 2: **CHEST FLY**

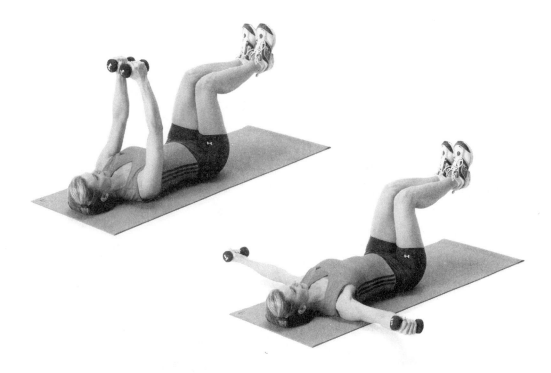

In Phase 1, you did chest flies with your feet on the mat. To increase the challenge for Phase 2, you'll do the same exercise with your legs raised. If you would like an even greater challenge, try it with your hips raised, forming a bridge with your body by pressing your feet into the floor, lifting your hips, and balancing on your shoulder blades.

For the version shown, lie with your back on the mat, with your knees bent and your feet on the mat. Lift your lower legs and bend your knees, forming a right angle. Firm your abs and tuck your tailbone. Extend your arms so your hands are above your chest with your elbows slightly bent.

Open your arms to the sides. Squeeze through your chest as you bring your hands back together, as if you were hugging someone tightly. Repeat for 1 minute.

1-MINUTE ABS

PHASE 1: **PILATES BICYCLE**

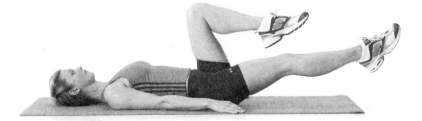

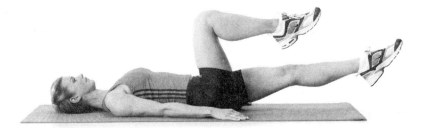

Lie with your back on a mat. Bring your left knee in toward your chest. Extend your right leg, lifting your foot about 12" off the floor. Pull your tummy to your spine.

Keeping your tummy firm, switch legs, extending your left leg and bringing your right leg toward your chest. Continue switching legs for 1 minute.

PHASE 2: **PILATES BICYCLE**

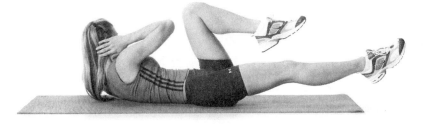

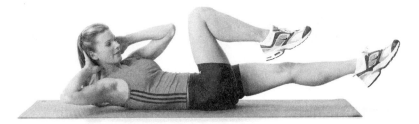

Lie with your back on a mat. Place your hands behind your head, elbows open to the sides. Bring your left knee in toward your chest. Extend your right leg, lifting your foot about 12" off the floor. Lift your head, neck, and shoulders off the mat and pull your tummy to your spine.

Keeping your tummy firm, switch legs, extending your left leg and bringing your right leg toward your chest while bringing your left elbow toward your right knee. Continue switching legs for 1 minute.

The 3-2-1 Buns Circuit

This fun sports-inspired circuit will keep you mentally entertained as you dribble, kick, and shoot. The squats during the strength training will help to lift and shape your backside. Training this large muscle will also add more power to your step. You'll feel better able to bound up steps or trudge up a hill. Finally, the reverse curls during the abdominal circuit will help to strengthen the lower part of the tummy, below the belly button—another common trouble spot, especially if you've ever had a baby.

3-MINUTE CARDIO

PHASES 1 and 2: STEP TOUCH WITH A SOCCER KICK

FOR PHASE 1: Starting with your feet wider than hip-distance apart, step your right foot toward your left, bending your knees slightly as you do so.

Step your right foot back to its starting position.

Pretend to kick a soccer ball with your right foot, aiming the ball 45 degrees to the left. Keep your right leg extended as you kick, connecting with the ball with the side of your foot. Return your foot to the starting position, repeating the entire sequence for 30 seconds before switching kicking legs.

FOR PHASE 2: Do the exercise as described in Phase 1, but to increase the intensity, add a hop to the move as you return your feet to the starting position.

PHASES 1 AND 2: **SHOOT A BASKETBALL**

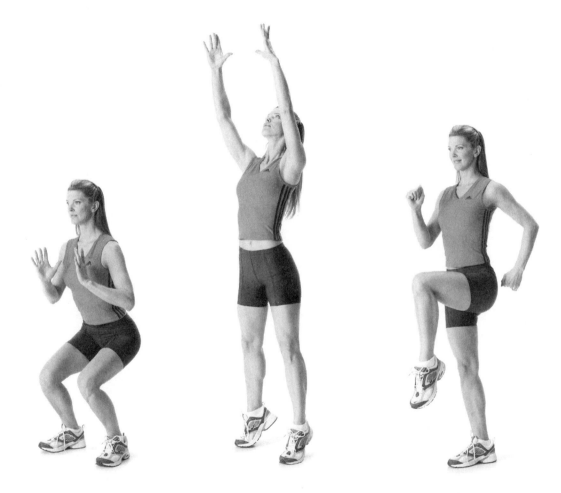

FOR BOTH PHASES: Bend your knees and squat down. As you do so, pretend you are holding a basketball at chest level, with your arms in front of your chest and your elbows bent.

All in one motion, extend your legs, jump, and shoot, thrusting your arms overhead.

Land (making sure to bend your knees) and march in place for a few steps before repeating the sequence. Continue to shoot hoops for 1 minute. For a lower-intensity version, keep your toes on the ground, lifting only your heels during the jumping part of the move.

PHASES 1 AND 2: **CATCH A FOOTBALL**

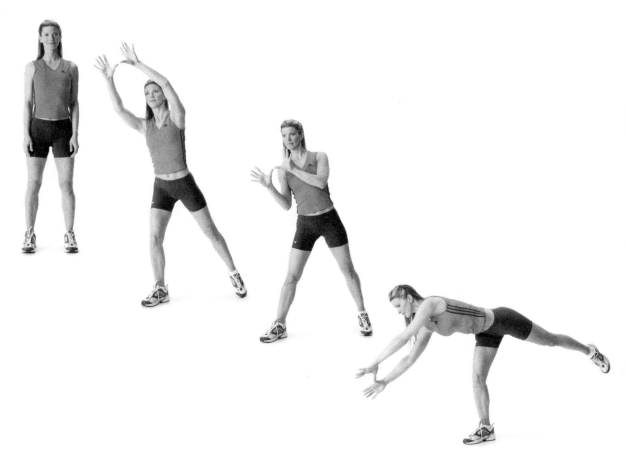

FOR BOTH PHASES: Start with your feet slightly wider than hip distance apart and your knees slightly bent. Pretend someone is tossing a football to you, with the ball coming in about a foot above and to the outside of your right shoulder. To catch the ball, you must step to the right and then jump into the air, raising your arms to get the ball.

Land with your knees slightly bent, then repeat, this time fielding a ball at chest level.

Land again with your knees slightly bent, then repeat, this time catching the ball around knee level. Alternate between the three movements for 30 seconds before switching sides. For a lower-intensity version, keep your toes on the ground, lifting only your heels during the jumping part of the move.

2-MINUTE STRENGTHENING

PHASE 1: SQUAT WITH LEG LIFT

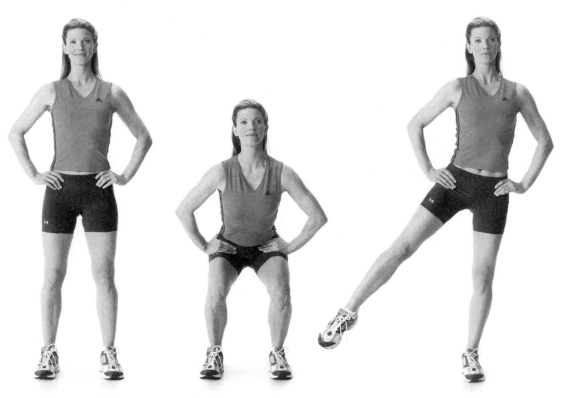

Starting with your feet slightly more than hip distance apart, bend your knees and squat down, keeping your chest lifted as you squat. Lower slowly, counting 3-2-1 as you do so. As you extend your legs to rise, squeeze your buns.

Shift your body weight over your left foot as you lift your right leg out to the side. Lower your right leg, squat, and rise, this time lifting your left leg out to the side. Continue squatting and alternately lifting your legs for 1 minute.

PHASE 2: **SQUAT WITH LEG LIFT**

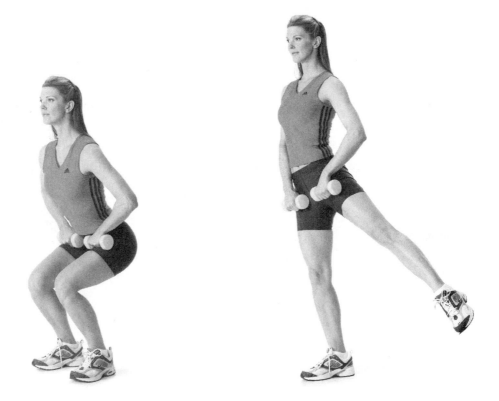

Grasp a light dumbbell in each hand and place your hands at the tops of your thighs. Starting with your feet slightly wider than hip distance apart, bend your knees and squat down, keeping your chest lifted as you squat. Lower slowly, counting 3-2-1 as you do so.

Shift your body weight over your right foot as you lift your left leg out to the side. Lower your left leg, squat, and rise, this time lifting your right leg to the side. Continue squatting and alternately lifting your legs for 1 minute.

PHASE 1: **SQUAT WITH KNEE LIFT**

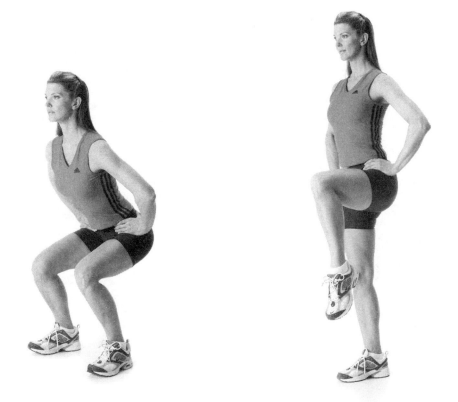

Starting with your feet slightly wider than hip distance apart, bend your knees and squat down, keeping your chest lifted as you squat. Lower slowly, counting 3-2-1 as you do so.

Extend your legs to rise, squeezing your buns. When you're standing, lift your left knee toward your chest. Hold for 1 second, then lower your foot to the floor. Squat and then lift your right knee toward your chest. Continue alternating legs for 1 minute.

PHASE 2: **SQUAT WITH FRONT KICK**

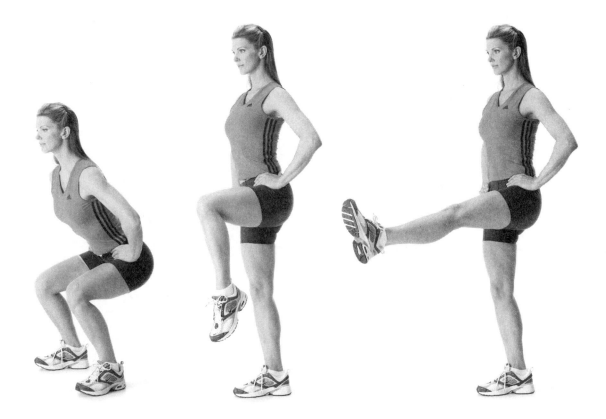

Place your hands on your hips with your elbows bent. Starting with your feet slightly wider than hip distance apart, bend your knees and squat down, keeping your chest lifted as you squat. Lower slowly, counting 3-2-1 as you do so.

Extend your legs to rise, squeezing your buns. When you're standing, lift your right knee toward your chest and then kick it forward. Hold for 1 second, then lower your foot to the floor. Squat, then stand and lift your left knee toward your chest for a front kick. Continue for 1 minute, alternating legs.

1-MINUTE ABS

PHASES 1 AND 2: **REVERSE CURL WITH TOE REACH**

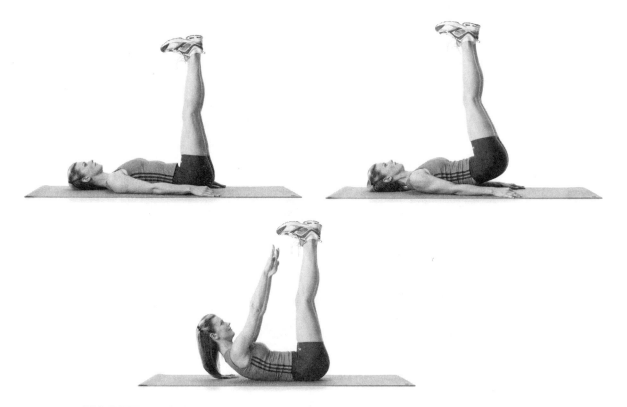

FOR BOTH PHASES: Lie on your back and lift your legs toward the ceiling so they form a 90-degree angle with your torso. Rest your arms at your sides, palms facing down.

Exhale as you lift your feet toward the ceiling, bringing your tailbone and hips off the mat. Lower and repeat this step for 30 seconds.

Keeping your legs extended toward the ceiling, stretch your hands toward your toes, lifting your head, shoulders, and upper back off the floor as you do so. Lower and repeat for 30 seconds. For a lower-intensity version, keep your legs bent so that your knees are at a 90-degree angle as you bring your tailbone off the mat.

The 3-2-1 Back Circuit

You will dance your way through this fun circuit, almost forgetting for a moment that you are exercising and burning calories! The double arm rows and back extensions you will complete during the strengthening phase help to strengthen your upper and lower back. The rows target the typically weak muscles between the shoulder blades. Strengthening them will help you to stand taller, which will make you appear slimmer. The back extensions strengthen your lower back, helping to prevent back pain. Finally; the body plank strengthens a deep abdominal muscle called the *transverse abdominus*. This muscle acts like a girdle for your entire midsection; strengthening it helps to naturally pull in your center so you will appear slimmer.

3-MINUTE CARDIO

PHASES 1 AND 2: MAMBO

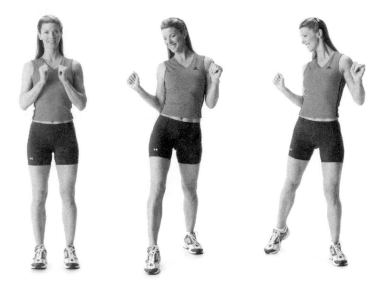

FOR BOTH PHASES: Start with your feet under your hips. Step your right foot forward to 2 o'clock, thrusting your right hip outward as you do so. As you step, circle your arms toward each other (toward the midline of your torso), then overhead and out.

Next, step back to 5 o'clock, again thrusting your hip outward. As you step, circle your arms downward, bringing them down the midline of your torso and then out to the sides. Have fun with this sensual Latin dance! Repeat for 30 seconds, then switch sides for another 30 seconds.

PHASES 1 and 2: **POWER SQUAT**

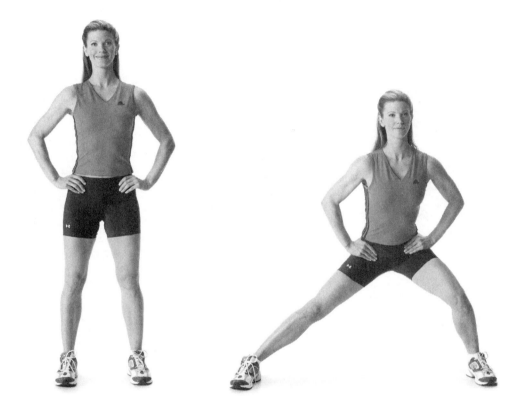

FOR PHASE 1: Start with your feet under your hips and your hands on your hips.

Take a large step to the right (as large a step as you can take). Squat down as far as you comfortably can, stopping once your thighs are parallel with the floor, then rise. Repeat for 30 seconds on the right, then switch sides and repeat for another 30 seconds.

FOR PHASE 2: Do the move as described in Phase 1, but to increase the intensity, instead of stepping to the right, hop your feet out to the sides before beginning the squat.

PHASES 1 and 2: **V-STEP**

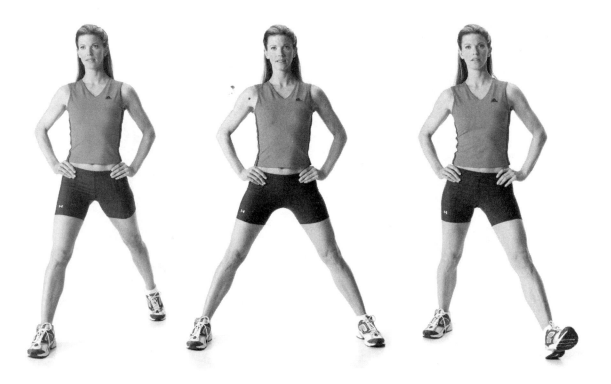

FOR PHASE 1: Pretend someone has drawn a large V on the floor. Start with your feet under your hips at the bottom of the V. Step your right foot to the top right end of the V.

Step your left foot to the top left end of the V.

Step your right foot to the starting position, then follow with your left. Continue stepping to each corner of the V for 1 minute.

FOR PHASE 2: Do the move as described in Phase 1, but to increase the intensity, try hopping into position instead of stepping. Keep your movements smooth and under control.

2-MINUTE STRENGTHENING

PHASE 1: DOUBLE ARM ROW

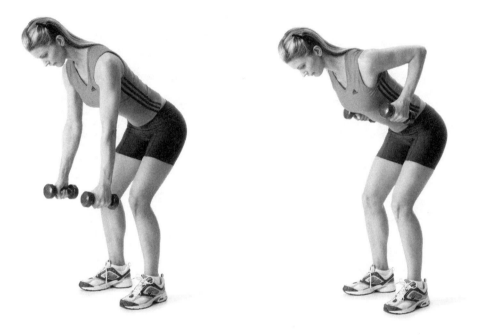

Stand with your feet under your hips and grasp a light dumbbell in each hand. Bend your knees slightly, bend forward from the hips at about 45 degrees, and extend your arms.

Bend your elbows, keeping them close to your torso as you row with your "paddles," bringing your elbows as far behind your back as you can. Squeeze your shoulder blades as you do so, as if you were trying to squeeze a pencil between them. Return to the starting position and repeat for 1 minute.

PHASE 2: **DOUBLE ARM ROW**

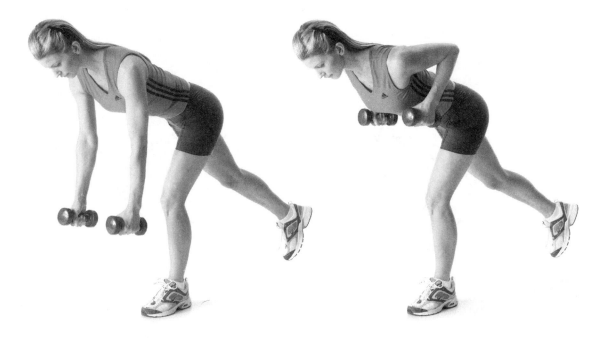

Do the exercise as described in Phase 1, but to increase the intensity, use heavier weights or balance on one leg as you complete the movement.

PHASES 1 and 2: **BACK EXTENSION**

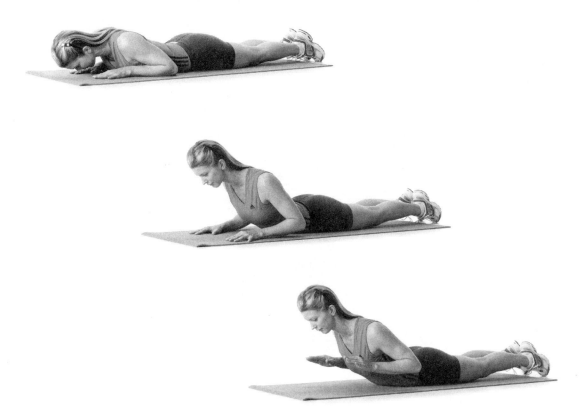

FOR PHASE 1: Lie on your tummy with your legs extended, the tops of your feet against the floor, your elbows bent, and your palms on the floor on either side of your chin. Keeping your elbows close to your body and using your arms as little as possible, use your back muscles to lift your head, shoulders, and back. Hold for 1 second, then lower. Repeat for 1 minute. Keep your abs firm throughout the exercise.

FOR PHASE 2: Do the exercise as described in Phase 1, except place your hands under your chin.

1-MINUTE ABS

PHASE 1: **BODY PLANK**

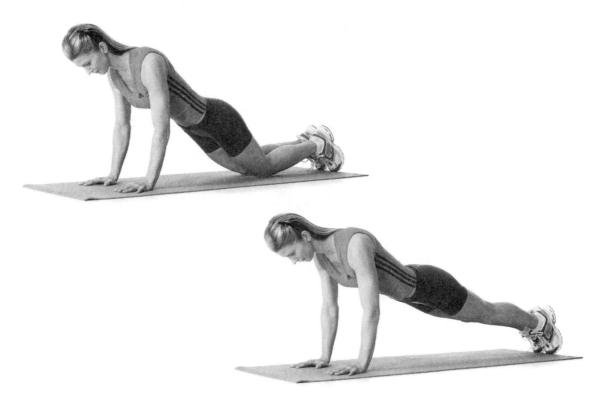

Kneel with your feet and knees on the floor. Lean forward and place your hands on the floor under your shoulders. Lean your body weight into your hands and straighten your legs, forming a straight, diagonal line from your knees to your head. Scoop your tummy inward and hold for 1 minute.

PHASE 2: **BODY PLANK**

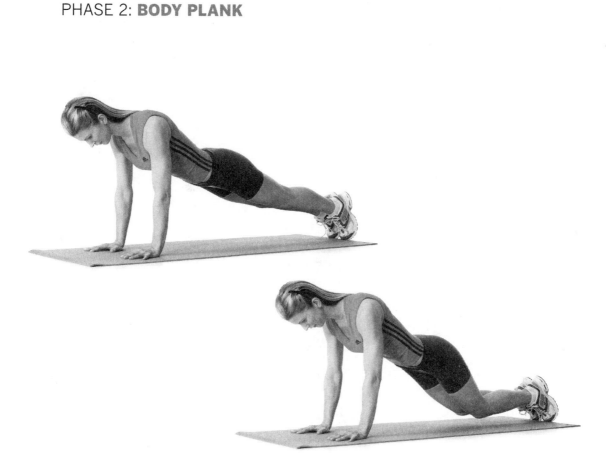

Come into a pushup position with your hands under your chest and your legs extended.
Lengthen your entire body, reaching back through your heels and forward through the
top of your head.

Slowly lower your knees to the floor (but do not touch it), counting 3-2-1 as you do so.
Raise your knees, then repeat lowering and raising for 1 minute.

The 3-2-1 Cooldown

The following cooldown for both Phase 1 and Phase 2 includes stretches for your legs and shoulders. In particular, you will stretch body areas that are unusually tight for most women. Move into each stretch slowly and breathe into the sensation of the stretch. Breathing will help you to relax, which enables your muscle to relax and lengthen. Feel free to add your own favorite stretches to this routine and change the stretches periodically. The most important thing is that you stretch after your workout—so do the stretches you like!

SHOULDER STRETCH

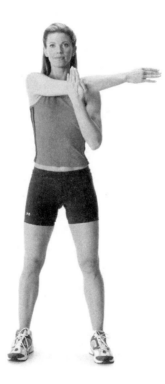

Stand with your feet slightly wider than shoulder distance apart. Bring your right arm across your chest, using your left hand to gently pull your arm in to increase the stretch to the back of your shoulder. Hold for 15 to 20 seconds. Repeat with the other arm.

STANDING CALF STRETCH

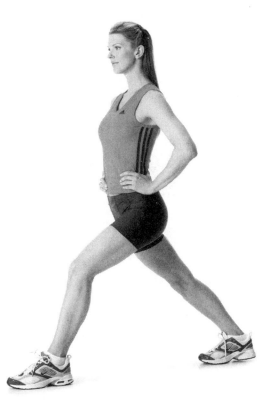

Bring your legs into a scissor position, with your left foot about 2½' in front of your right. Place your hands on your hips. Push into the floor with both feet until you feel a stretch in the calf of your back leg. Hold for 15 to 20 seconds. Switch legs and repeat.

RUNNER'S STRETCH

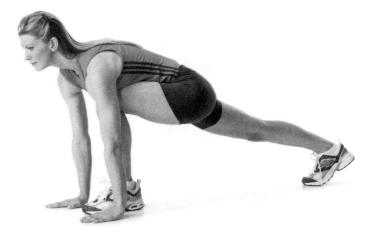

Bring your legs into a scissor position, with your left foot about $2\frac{1}{2}'$ in front of your right. Bend your left knee and lean forward, bringing the front of your torso near your thigh and placing your fingertips or palms against the floor (depending on your flexibility). Allow your right heel to rise, but keep your leg extended. Reach back through your right foot and forward through your left knee, allowing your pubic bone to drop downward. Hold for 15 to 20 seconds. Switch legs and repeat.

QUAD STRETCH

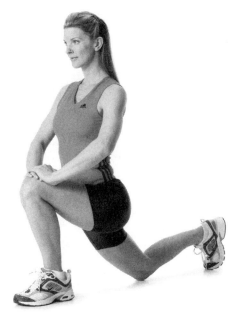

From the runner's stretch with your left leg forward, bend your right knee and place it on the floor. Lift your torso until it is upright. Place your hands against your left knee for support. Bend your right knee and lift your right foot. If flexibility allows, grasp your right foot with your right hand. If you cannot grasp your foot, just lift it until you feel a stretch. Hold it for 15 to 20 seconds. Switch legs and repeat.

HAMSTRING STRETCH

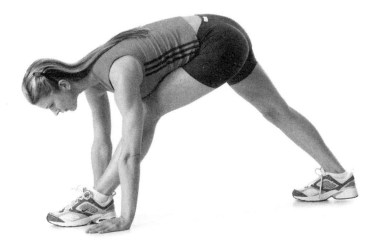

From the quad stretch with your left leg forward, lower your right foot to the floor. Straighten your left leg, reach back through your hips, and bend forward, bringing your face toward your left knee, placing your fingertips or palms on the floor for support, and pointing your left foot. Hold for 15 to 20 seconds. Switch legs and repeat.

3·2·1
SUCCESS STORY
Earnestine Cole

Age: 50+

Accomplishment: Lost 11 pounds in five weeks, reduced systolic blood pressure by 14 points and diastolic by 18 points, and dropped from a size 1X to a size 18

Q: How did you gain the excess weight?

A: I led a busy life until now and did not give any thought to what I ate or how little I slept. I'm a journalist, and at times, when working on projects, I would stay up for two-day stretches with just a couple of hours of sleep. The stress and my poor eating habits added 135 pounds to my body over the years.

Q: How does this weight loss plan compare to others you have tried?

A: I have tried Jenny Craig, the South Beach Diet, and the Atkins Diet. I've also exercised with three personal fitness trainers. On this plan, eating was no problem for me. For me, food is food—always delicious! I got full and had no hunger cravings after the first week on the program. This plan called for nutritious, healthy meals and snacks. After Week 1, I wasn't tempted to overeat, nor did I crave food. None of the other diets or exercise programs worked for me like this one.

Q: What changes have you noticed in your physical health?

A: When I first started 3-2-1, I felt tired, depressed, and defeated. I thought I was in way over my head! After Week 1, my energy level increased, and the tiredness during the daytime left my body. I felt like doing more things more often, such as cooking and cleaning. My concentration improved, and I found that I wasn't always forgetting things.

Q: How do you feel about 3-2-1 exercise?

A: The workout does exactly what it promised—it put me on the road to better health. I felt challenged from Day 1, which was a surprise for me as I had been working out five days a week for two years. I thought the 3-2-1 workout would be simple and easy, not much work for me. I'm so glad I was wrong! At the end of the workout, I was breathless and sweaty. After the fourth workout, however, the sessions got easier. I felt challenged when I started the workout and successful at the end of it because I hung in there until I completed the last exercise.

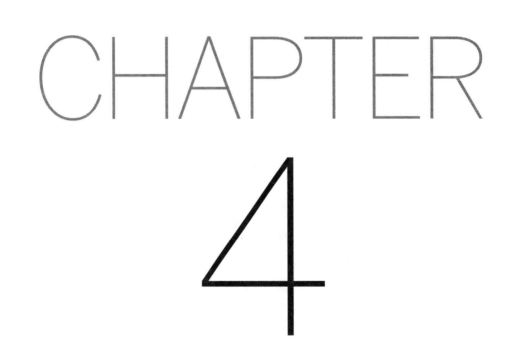

CHAPTER

4

3·2·1 MOTIVATION

DAILY STRATEGIES THAT ENSURE YOUR SUCCESS

In your hands, you are holding the most effective solutions to your weight loss struggles. The 3-2-1 eating plan and the 3-2-1 fitness plan will help you lose weight and feel good while you are doing it. Your 3-2-1 meal plan includes the opportunity for a daily treat to help reduce the feeling of deprivation that often leads to cheating, overeating, and abandoning a diet before you've reached your goal. The 3-2-1 exercise plan enables you to feel confident and in control, which in turn puts you in a positive mindset to help you follow through with 3-2-1 eating.

For lasting success, however, you need more. I tell all of my clients that successful weight loss is 50 percent attitude. You need more than just great diet and exercise plans. You also need mental strategies that will help you follow those plans. Like any achievement—and weight loss is a big achievement—losing weight requires constant effort, positive thinking, patience, and discipline. That's what 3-2-1 motivation is all about.

Weight loss is hard work. Yet, if you stick with it, your efforts pay off in huge dividends. A smaller clothing size, better health, more energy, improved self-esteem, and reduced preoccupation with food are well worth all of your struggles.

■

Weight loss and weight maintenance is a continual, lifelong project. The effort you put into the project is well worth it, but you can only win this battle if you see it clearly for what it is—an ongoing assignment. So before you start, I want you to commit, right now, to starting 3-2-1 and following it to completion. Sure, you might slip up along the way. You might go out to eat instead of cooking a 3-2-1 dinner one night. You might take a nap, go out with friends, or find any number of other excuses to skip a 3-2-1 workout on a particular day.

No matter how you stray from the plan over the course of the next few weeks, months, or years, commit yourself this very minute to getting right back on track as soon as you're able (optimally, at the next meal or on the next day). You've failed only if you view falling off the wagon as the end of your program. So decide to do it, stick with it, and follow through. Make eating well and exercising your number one priority for as long as it takes you to lose weight. It's important to your health, your well-being, and your loved ones.

DAILY MOTIVATORS

Take steps to motivate yourself every day. In the following pages, you will find some easy and straightforward strategies to accomplish that goal. You don't need to incorporate all of them into your life, but try to keep an open mind and consider which ones might help you over the coming weeks as you start your 3-2-1 nutrition and exercise plans.

3 ▪ Three (or More) Times a Day

Link the following strategies with your meals and snacks, using them between three and six times a day.

Close each meal with a ritual. Chewing and eating give us pleasure, which is why you may have a tendency to extend the pleasure of eating long after you have satisfied your physical hunger (and may actually become quite uncomfortably full). If you tend to serve yourself second and third helpings or to continually walk back to the kitchen or office break room in search of snacks, you will need to find a different way to satisfy your urge to chew. Many of my clients have broken their dependence on grazing by closing their meals with a ritual. The following rituals help to psychologically reinforce the concept that once the meal is over, it's time to move on to other tasks. When you use one or more of them at the end of a meal or snack, you help to quiet the part of your mind that distracts you with thoughts about food, thus creating more mental energy for work, hobbies, and other tasks. Without all of the "food noise" in your head, you'll find you are much more productive. Consider using any or all of the following strategies to add closure to your meals.

- Light a candle for your meal and blow it out once you've finished. This simple strategy effectively says, "The meal is over."

- Brush your teeth after meals. Besides creating a mentally reinforcing ritual, brushing your teeth offers two side benefits. The most obvious: You'll have healthier teeth and gums. The less obvious: Few foods taste appealing right after you've brushed, so you'll more easily keep yourself out of the kitchen. In fact, a Japanese study of more than 14,000 people, published in the *Journal of the Japan Society for the Study of Obesity,* determined that people who brush after meals tend to weigh less than people who don't.

This strategy worked well for Jane, who suffered from night-eating syndrome. Jane often ate more than half of her daily calories at night, many of them as postdinner snacks. To break out of this cycle, she not only brushed and flossed after dinner, she also placed whitening strips on her teeth. To work effectively, the strips had to remain on her teeth for 30 minutes, and Jane couldn't drink or eat anything while she had them on. Once she removed them, she often found food unappealing. After 10 days of using this strategy, she not only was thinner and more in control of her nighttime eating, she also had beautiful white teeth!

• Chew sugarless gum after meals. This will keep your mouth busy and provide prolonged flavor for your taste buds without extra calories. In addition, chewing a stick of sugarless gum after a meal can help loosen and remove leftover food debris. (Of course, if you have the time or opportunity to brush, even better!)

• Drink a cup of hot tea. Choose any tea you like (including herbal, chamomile, black, green, oolong, peppermint, and ginger). Because it's hot, you'll have to slowly sip it over a long period of time, which takes your mind off eating. It also helps you to lengthen the pleasure of a meal without consuming calories.

ASK**JOY**

Will Gum Make Me Hungry?

Some weight loss Web sites tell you to avoid chewing gum at all costs. These sites claim that chewing stimulates the production of digestive enzymes, which make you feel hungry. This simply isn't true (unless, of course, you're already hungry before chewing the gum). Contrary to what many people think, sugarless gum does not stimulate your appetite. In fact, it's a great way to prevent yourself from popping something caloric in your mouth. So keep a pack of sugarless gum or breath mints on hand at all times.

Pay attention to your food. Do you multitask while eating? Perhaps you pay bills with a pen in one hand and a sandwich in the other, eat dinner in front of the television, or munch in front of your computer. If you do, know that these types of distractions can easily cause you to overeat. These tasks distract you from what you are doing, reducing the satisfaction of eating as well as causing you to ignore your natural physical cues to stop eating. In a study published in the journal *Physiology & Behavior*, 37 participants ate a buffet-style lunch in various settings, including while watching television. Eating while watching television increased food consumption by 14 percent. Other research has shown that people can more easily lose weight if they focus on the process of eating—the flavor, texture, and smell of their food—rather than distracting themselves with reading material or the television.

As a side benefit, eating meals at your dinner table may enable you to grow closer to your dining companions, especially your children. It also increases the chances that your children will grow up with a healthy attitude toward food. A study published in the journal *Appetite* found that teens who lived in homes where eating together was a priority and where meals took place in a positive, structured setting (such as at a table) were less likely to develop eating disorders than teens whose families did not prioritize eating together.

Pay attention to your sensations of hunger and fullness. Eat slowly and try to notice the earliest hints of fullness. Halfway through your meal, stop and rate your hunger on a scale from 1 to 5 (with 1 being ravenous and 5 being completely full). Try to stop eating at 3 or 4, when you feel comfortably full and satisfied.

Write down what you eat as you eat it. I probably am not the first person to suggest that you keep a food log, and I probably won't be the last. Study after study shows that keeping a food log—writing down what you eat when you eat it—helps you motivate yourself to lose weight and keep it off. When you write down what you eat, you have an easier time monitoring what you eat. In fact, many people find that keeping a food log causes them to eat differently—even if they are not following a formal diet. It makes them more conscious about every eating decision they make.

I've also found that many of my clients consume more extracurricular calories (calories not accounted for on a meal plan) than they realize. Once they start keeping a food log, they can see in black and white the soft drinks, condiments, and little nibbles here and there that add up over the course of a day.

I know you may be already planning to skip this piece of advice. I'll make a deal with you. Keep a log for the first three days of the 3-2-1 meal plan, writing down what you eat just after you eat it. (Don't wait until the end of the day to write down this information; you may forget about many of the little nibbles and indiscretions by then.) At the end of each day, look over your log and see how closely you stuck to the meal plan. This can really be motivating, as you'll have a record of just how hard you worked during the day.

After three days, stop keeping the log if you find the process more cumbersome than helpful. If you got a lot of benefit from the activity, however, consider keeping it up. You might also consider returning to logging your intake during typically challenging times for you, such as the holiday season or during a vacation. In one study, published in the journal *Health Psychology*, researchers determined that only people who kept detailed food records were able to lose weight over the holidays, whereas people who did not keep these records tended to gain weight over the same time period.

How do you keep your food log? That's up to you. Use a piece of paper, your personal data assistant, or a little notebook. Choose a log that you can carry with you at all times, so you can write down what you eat or drink immediately, while you still remember.

2 ▪ Twice a Day

I've found that few people overeat at breakfast. If anything, most people either skip it or undereat. Lunch and dinner, on the other hand (particularly dinner), can feel more challenging. The following tips will help you to more easily stick to your 3-2-1 meal plan during these important meals.

Drink two glasses of water before eating. You may have heard that water blunts your appetite or speeds your metabolism. Disregard that information. There is no magical or proven physiological weight loss effect to drinking water. Despite popular belief, downing a glass or two of water probably does not reduce your appetite very much, and any metabolism boost you get from drinking cold water is minimal at best. All of that said, drinking two glasses of water before your meal slows you down, preventing you from rushing right into the act of eating. It also makes your meal into a ritual. When you start your meal with two glasses of water, you go into your meal with a positive "I can do this" mindset. You followed plan A, which was drinking the water, so you feel more confident in following plan B, eating only the food on your plate—and no more.

As a side benefit, your two glasses of water will make you much less likely to reach for more diet-busting types of liquid calories. Liquids can often amount to a lot of extra calories that won't fill you up. You'll want to pass on soda, fruit drinks, fruit juice, smoothies, and coffee loaded with milk and sugar. When you drink a lot of water, you don't feel as thirsty and, as a result, don't feel tempted to reach for caloric beverages.

Health bonus: Guzzling two glasses of water before lunch and dinner will help you meet your daily fluid requirement. And water is needed to help move along all the fiber-rich food you'll be eating.

If you don't like the taste of water, think of it as health medicine. One of my clients even held her nose when she first began drinking her two glasses before meals. After a while, she grew to actually enjoy it. Do whatever works for you!

Slow down and enjoy the moment. People who gobble down their food tend to consume more overall calories than people who eat at a leisurely pace. When you eat too quickly, you may miss the natural body cues that tell you that your body no longer needs calories. Consequently, you overeat and end up feeling stuffed. No matter how quickly you eat right now, you can take steps to slow down. The easiest way to slow down is to try to take in what you eat through all of your senses. Usually, most people use only the sense of taste when eating—and if you eat very quickly, you may eat a lot of your food without actually experiencing it. Instead, try doing the following at lunch and dinner (particularly dinner).

- Look at your food. Notice the color and texture.

- Smell your food before you eat it. Experience the wonderful sensation of smelling delicious food when you are hungry.

- Take a bite and notice the texture of the food in your mouth. Is it smooth? Chewy? Crunchy?

- Sip water after every few bites—and even put your fork down.

Continue to notice your food as the meal progresses. You may find that the food looks, smells, and tastes *most* appealing at the beginning of the meal, with the pleasure of eating diminishing over the course of the meal.

1 ▪ Once a Day, Once a Week

At the end of the day and end of the week, you may benefit from carving out a little time for yourself to regroup and look at the day (or week) that you just finished, along with the day (or week) ahead. During this preparatory time, consider doing the following.

Look over your food log. At the end of the day, reviewing your log can help you feel good about everything you've done *right*. If you keep your log long term, you might use this time to also solve problems. Consider writing additional factors into your log, beyond just the food that you ate. You might, for example, keep notes on your emotional state before meals, your exercise sessions (Did you complete the entire routine? Did you feel energized or tired?), and the type of day you had in general (Were you stressed? Relaxed? Busy?). These notes will help you to see if you tend to stray from your meal plan or overeat when you are under stress or if you turn to food to soothe negative emotions. You might also be able to spot patterns in your eating—

for example, a late-afternoon or late-evening nibbling habit. Once you have this information, you can more easily go into these situations with the right mindset and strategy.

Plan your meals. Take 10 minutes every evening to look at your meal plan for the following day. (Or, at the very latest, do it in the morning before you start the day.) Make sure you have the foods you will need on hand, that your day will allow you the time to cook, and that the meals meet your personal standards for foods you (or your family) like to eat. You don't have to religiously follow the order of the 3-2-1 meal plan. You can mix and match various lunches and dinners as needed. So if you find you have a busy day and need to prepare a low-fuss meal, flip through the plan and find something that meets your needs. This small amount of planning time will help prevent you from coming up with a much less weight loss–friendly solution in the heat of the moment—such as ordering pizza or eating fast food.

Once a week, look over the plan and designate this day as your grocery shopping day. Although you may like to pick up certain foods as you need them, I can guarantee that you will increase your chances of sticking to the meal plan if you have most of what you need on hand at the beginning of the week. It's all too easy to give yourself the excuse to eat out when you don't feel like running to the store at the last minute to buy a particular ingredient.

Pre-portion your snacks. There's no chance of overeating when you have only one portion in front of you. Try the following single-serving snacks when you want something fun to eat: Skinny Cow frozen desserts, 100-calorie snack packs, Pria bars, Tootsie Pop lollipops, Edy's Fruit Bars, and Swiss Miss fat-free pudding.

Check in with a support person. Study after study shows that you can more easily lose weight and keep it off if you have support than if you try to go it alone. A supportive friend can help you to solve problems, listen to you vent frustrations (so they don't cause you to turn to food), and even increase your confidence. So consider lining up at least one person to support you in your efforts. You might choose a close friend, your spouse, someone at your gym, or even an online buddy you met in a weight loss discussion group. At the end of each day, check in with your support person. Brag about your successes: the weight you've lost, the recipes you've prepared, the new exercises you've tried, the meal plan you stuck to religiously, the cravings you overcame, and so on. Also, use this time to complain and vent about your weight loss–related frustrations. Unload your anger about all the hard work ("It's not fair!") and your anxiety about the future ("I'm not sure I can keep it up!"). Talk about particularly hard times during the day and work with your support person to solve problems that might stand in the way of success.

End each day on a positive note. No matter how you ate or exercised on any given day, you've worked hard and put in a good effort. So give yourself a pat on the back for having a productive day. Notice what you've done right and congratulate yourself for your effort.

YOUR JUST REWARDS

I started this chapter with a warning, making sure you knew about the hard work you have ahead. Now I want to provide an alternative view. Yes, weight loss is hard, but it's also incredibly rewarding. As you lose weight, you will feel better physically, feel more confident, and have more energy. You'll also feel more comfortable moving, walking, working, and playing.

When and if the going gets tough, try to focus on these payoffs. You're energetic. You're in control. You're satisfied. Isn't your hard work worth it for the outcome? Isn't it

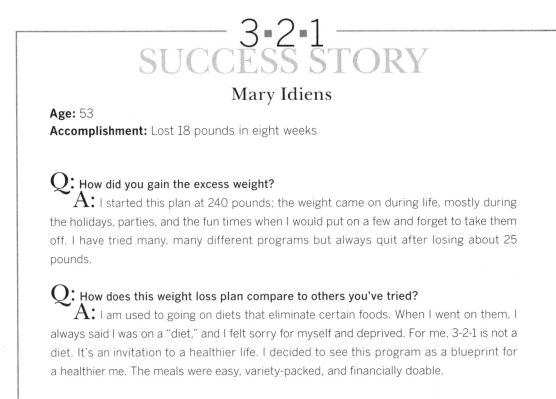

3·2·1 SUCCESS STORY

Mary Idiens

Age: 53
Accomplishment: Lost 18 pounds in eight weeks

Q: How did you gain the excess weight?
A: I started this plan at 240 pounds; the weight came on during life, mostly during the holidays, parties, and the fun times when I would put on a few and forget to take them off. I have tried many, many different programs but always quit after losing about 25 pounds.

Q: How does this weight loss plan compare to others you've tried?
A: I am used to going on diets that eliminate certain foods. When I went on them, I always said I was on a "diet," and I felt sorry for myself and deprived. For me, 3-2-1 is not a diet. It's an invitation to a healthier life. I decided to see this program as a blueprint for a healthier me. The meals were easy, variety-packed, and financially doable.

worth it for better health, increased energy, and a more slender and fit body?

More important, isn't it worth it to wake up in the morning and not feel bloated or guilty from what you ate the night before? Isn't it worth it for the peace of mind you will soon have because you no longer worry about every bite of food you put in your mouth? Isn't it worth it to feel comfortable in your own skin? Isn't it worth it to look in the mirror and like the person you see staring back at you? Isn't it worth it for the realization that you've accomplished something big, a project few people have the courage not only to start but also to complete?

Make weight loss your marathon. Yes, you'll sweat. You'll work hard. But you'll also get that medal—the new and improved body—at the finish line. You'll find that one day, you will look back on all of this, and you will confidently say to yourself, "I'm so glad I did this. I feel so great about myself now." Yes, you will work hard every day for the rest of your life, but you'll feel proud of your hard work and proud of the body that your hard work created.

Q: What changes have you noticed in your physical health?
A: I have more energy, less shortness of breath, and a more positive attitude. I feel alive and ready to conquer. I now treat myself as a valuable commodity that deserves to eat healthy and that deserves time out for physical activity.

Q: What do you think of the exercise?
A: Working out daily has become a way of life. If I don't do any exercise by 4:00 p.m., I feel restless. I do 3-2-1 at least every other day.

Q: How do your hunger and cravings fare on this compared to others you've tried?
A: The first week was the hardest. I had to stop myself from wanting to go out and just grab anything. I also had to adjust to measuring my portions. That took a bit of focusing. After the first week, however, I did not feel I was on a diet. I felt I was just eating healthier.

Q: What was your overall experience with 3-2-1?
A: It was totally positive. Three meals and two snacks is the way to go! It's how life should be.

CHAPTER

5

YOUR COUNTDOWN TO SUCCESS

WEIGHT LOSS GOALS THAT ALLOW YOU TO LOVE YOUR BODY—AND LOVE LIVING IN YOUR BODY

You're almost ready to start eating, exercising, and thinking your way to a smaller body. Before you get started, however, let's take some time to set short-term and long-term goals. The goals you set today will help fuel your motivation tomorrow.

You may already have a goal in mind. For instance, you may have a dress or pair of jeans in your closet that you can't wait to be able to wear. You may have a number on the scale that you want to see. You may have a photo of yourself from many years ago and want to get back the body you had then.

There's nothing wrong with any of those goals, assuming they are realistic for you, your age, your metabolism, and your genetics. Goal setting requires a careful balance of optimism—believing that you can lose all the weight you want—and realism—choosing a weight loss destination that allows you to live sanely. If you pick a weight that's too low for your body, you're setting the stage to become obsessed with restricting food and overexercising to stay at that weight.

That's no way to live, which is why, in this chapter, you will learn how to set balanced, realistic goals—goals that allow you to look *and* feel great, goals that allow you to love your body but also love living in your body. What's realistic for you? That's hard to determine, and only you can know for sure. While making that determination, certainly keep in mind that the weight or body you had in high school or college may no longer be realistic for you today, especially if you are older than age 40. You can look fantastic after 40, but metabolism slows with age—especially after menopause. To reach and maintain the weight of your youth, you might have to eat much less food than you did 15 years ago.

Don't get me wrong. You are capable of anything, really anything. I've worked with people who have lost startling amounts of weight—25 pounds, 50 pounds, 100 pounds, and more—and have kept it off, all the while doing manageable amounts of exercise and following a sound eating plan. Just make sure you set a realistic goal and keep things in perspective.

DEFINE YOUR DESTINATION

Soon I will give you some hints about determining a long-term goal, but I encourage you to think smaller and more short term. You might eventually want to lose 100 pounds, but large-number goals tend to be quite overwhelming. Instead, I'd like you to consider making your goal something more immediate, such as shooting for 10 pounds. Once you lose 10, you can, of course, lose 10 more and 10 more until you eventually lose all the weight you want.

You'll approach weight loss in the way that many runners approach training for and running a marathon. Rather than focus on the daunting 26.2 miles that they must traverse, many runners instead talk themselves through the race by focusing on getting to the next mile marker, the next tree, or the next curve in the road. Each time they achieve a small goal, they regroup and say, "Okay, I can keep going to the next mile marker, curve, tree, etc."

In this way, you might think of each 10-pound loss as a mile marker along your longer weight loss journey. Feel proud of yourself each time you pass one of these markers. You worked hard to get there!

If you are comfortable with setting smaller, shorter-term goals, you may not need to formulate a long-term goal. Enjoy the journey. You may not know your final destination, but each 10 pounds lost will confirm that you are indeed moving in the right direction!

If you are the type of person who absolutely needs to start with the end in mind, you may decide to keep track of your body mass index (BMI). A number of studies have used BMI to determine the healthiest weight for your height. To determine your BMI, divide your weight in pounds by your height in inches squared and multiply by 703. For example, if you weigh 150 pounds and stand 5' 5" (65") tall, you would calculate your BMI as follows.

$$[150/(65 \times 65)] \times 703 = 24.96$$

The following government Web sites will calculate your BMI for you:

www.cdc.gov/nccdphp/dnpa/bmi/index.htm

http://nhlbisupport.com/bmi/

HEIGHT	WEIGHT (LB)													
4'10"	91	96	100	105	110	115	119	124	129	134	138	143	148	153
4'11"	94	99	104	109	114	119	124	128	133	138	143	148	153	158
5'0"	97	102	107	112	118	123	128	133	138	143	148	153	158	163
5'1"	100	106	111	116	122	127	132	137	143	148	153	158	164	169
5'2"	104	109	115	120	126	131	136	142	147	153	158	164	169	175
5'3"	107	113	118	124	130	135	141	146	152	158	163	169	175	180
5'4"	110	116	122	128	134	140	145	151	157	163	169	174	180	186
5'5"	114	120	126	132	138	144	150	156	162	168	174	180	186	192
5'6"	118	124	130	136	142	148	155	161	167	173	179	186	192	198
5'7"	121	127	134	140	146	153	159	166	172	178	185	191	198	204
5'8"	125	131	138	144	151	158	164	171	177	184	190	197	203	210
5'9"	128	135	142	149	155	162	169	176	182	189	196	203	209	216
5'10"	132	139	146	153	160	167	174	181	188	195	202	209	216	222
5'11"	136	143	150	157	165	172	179	186	193	200	208	215	222	229
6'0"	140	147	154	162	169	177	184	191	199	206	213	221	228	235
BMI	19	20	21	22	23	24	25	26	27	28	29	30	31	32

A body mass index below 18.5 is considered underweight. A BMI between 18.5 and 24.9 is normal weight and is associated with the lowest risk of obesity-related health complications. A BMI between 25 and 29.9 indicates overweight, which increases your risk of disease. And finally, a BMI of 30 or higher is considered obese. The higher your number above 25, the greater your health risk. If you are extremely muscular (a factor that usually applies only to serious athletes), this may throw off your BMI. Do not use this method if you row crew or competitively race bicycles, or if you're a body builder or you do some other sport that puts on a great deal of muscle. Instead, go by your measurements or by how your clothes fit.

HOW TO KNOW IF YOU ARE MOVING IN THE RIGHT DIRECTION

If you picked a short-term or long-term (or both) weight loss goal, then you will get on the scale from time to time to see whether you are moving toward (or away from) your goal.

During the first two weeks of the plan, you will lose the most weight. You might even lose up to 10 pounds during this time. The amount will depend on how many pounds you have to lose and how much you were eating before you started. People who have a lot of weight to lose or who are eating large quantities of food will lose the most weight the most quickly. Some of this weight loss comes from losing water, not fat. Once you cut back on the calories that you consume, your body will release some water, and you will immediately feel lighter and less bloated. Even within a week, the scale might register a loss of up to 5 pounds.

This is uplifting, and it should be. Just don't expect to continue to lose at this pace. After the initial two weeks, your weight loss will balance out, and you can then expect to lose up to 1 percent of your body weight each week. For most people, that comes to between ½ pound and 2 pounds a week.

As you lose weight, the pounds will come off more slowly. In fact, your weight will plateau from time to time. This doesn't necessarily mean the program is not working or that you are not following the program correctly. You may experience a short-term plateau (of up to three weeks) because of any of the following factors.

Muscle gain. If you are out of shape, your 3-2-1 workouts will help you to strengthen and build muscle, which weighs more than fat. While following this program, you'll be swapping fat for muscle and perhaps see no results on the scale from time to time. You will, however, *see* the results when you look in the mirror or get dressed in the morning. Fat takes up more space than muscle, so a 145-pound woman with very little body fat and a lot of muscle will look much leaner and more slender than another 145-pound woman with more fat and less muscle.

Fluid retention. Your menstrual cycle, medication, or something you ate may cause you to retain fluid, which will temporarily affect your weight on the scale.

Bowel habits. From time to time, your bowel movements may change or become less frequent, which can affect your weight.

OTHER WAYS TO MONITOR YOUR PROGRESS

Because so many non–fat cell related variables can affect your weight on any given day, you may decide to use a backup method to monitor your progress. It will help you to keep temporary plateaus in perspective. Consider using any of the following criteria.

Clothing Size and Fit

Clothing size is perhaps one of the most motivating ways to gauge your progress. There's nothing quite like the realization that you must cinch your belt a notch tighter to keep your pants from falling down! There's also nothing quite like celebrating your weight loss by shopping for a new outfit in a smaller size.

Before you start 3-2-1, try on a few specific articles of clothing, especially items that you used to love but no longer wear because they fit too tightly. Perhaps you choose a favorite pair of jeans, a little black dress, and a pants suit you once loved. Try them on and notice exactly how they fit. Can you pull the pants above your thighs? Can you get the zipper all the way up? Where do the clothes hug your body too tightly?

Try on the same clothes once a week as you lose weight. Each week, notice how the clothing becomes looser and looser. Eventually, when it becomes too baggy to wear, go shopping for a smaller size.

If you use clothing fit and size to monitor your progress, keep in mind that dry cleaning and laundering can shrink clothing. Don't despair if your once-roomy jeans suddenly feel tight after you've washed them. If you've been following 3-2-1 word for word, chalk it up to the dryer effect. One day, those jeans will be roomy straight out of the dryer.

Measurements

Your measurements can prevent you from becoming discouraged when the scale doesn't budge. I've counseled plenty of women who didn't lose weight on the scale—sometimes for weeks—but continued to lose inches.

To track your measurements, take out a flexible tape measure and record the measurements of your upper arms, waist, hips, and upper thighs.

Do this once every two weeks, keeping notes in a notebook and comparing your results from week to week. You'll lose inches at different rates from different areas of your body. Some people lose from their waist first, whereas others lose from their thighs (sadly, we all lose from our bust!). Your genetics largely determine this, so don't get discouraged. Also, keep in mind that at certain times of the month, you will retain water (especially in your stomach), and this will throw off your measurements.

Body Fat

If you are very fit, your high amount of muscle mass may throw off typical height-weight chart calculations as well as body mass index. I've worked with some body builders, elite athletes, and other muscular folks who were technically obese by body mass index or height-weight chart standards but who were actually very lean, with only a minimal amount of body fat.

In this case, a more accurate gauge of your fitness and health may be your percentage of lean body mass (muscle, bone, and other nonfat tissues) compared to your percentage of body fat.

Although some manufacturers now sell inexpensive body fat scales, to get an absolutely accurate sense of your changing body composition, sign up for body composition testing at a local fitness center, hospital, or university body composition lab that offers these services to the public. Get your body composition tested once before you start and once a month thereafter.

Use any of the following methods for body fat testing.

Skin fold calipers. These look like a set of pliers and are used by a testing professional to pinch areas of your body. The professional will use the calipers to pinch and measure the thickness of the skin on your upper arms, lower stomach, and thighs. Results can vary from one tester to another. Look for someone who tests with calipers regularly and try to get the same tester each time you get your body fat tested. Also, don't get tested after exercise. It causes the skin to swell slightly, which will register as a higher percentage of body fat than you actually have.

Underwater weighing and the "BOD POD." These highly accurate ways to gauge your level of body fat require specialized equipment, so they are usually available only at universities and research institutions. For underwater weighing, you sit on a scale that is situated in a small pool of warm water. You blow air out of your lungs as the platform lowers you into the water. Once you are completely submerged (for about 5 seconds), your underwater weight registers on a digital scale. Then the technician uses a formula to determine your body composition based on the difference between your above-water and below-water weights.

The BOD POD is a newer body fat measuring device and, according to research, is somewhat less accurate than underwater weighing. To be measured, you wear a skin suit and sit inside an enclosed, egg-shaped container. The device measures your body volume, calculating it based on how much air your body displaces in the chamber. Using a calculation of your body volume and body weight, a technician can determine your body fat percentage.

Bioelectrical impedance. This is the type of measurement used in those inexpensive at-home body composition scales. A more effective way to use this technology, however, is to have a professional measure your body composition with electrodes or with a more sophisticated bioelectrical impedance scale. For the electrode method, the professional attaches one to your hand and another to your foot. If you use a scale, you step on it in bare feet. Either way, the foot pad or electrodes emit an electrical signal that travels through your body and back to the footpad or electrode. The faster the signal travels, the more muscle you have. The slower it travels, the more fat you have, as fat will block or slow down the signal. But some variables can throw off your reading. Both food in your stomach and dehydration can slow the signal, making your reading higher than it should be, so get tested on an empty stomach but after drinking a few glasses of water.

For women, 32 percent fat or higher is considered obese. Between 25 and 31 percent is considered acceptable, 21 to 24 percent is considered fit, and 14 to 20 percent is considered athletic. Try not to shoot for an arbitrary body fat percentage, as the optimal amount of body fat varies from woman to woman. Also, age plays a role, as you lose both muscle and bone mass as you age, making it harder to maintain a low body fat percentage.

READY TO LOSE?

Have you set a goal and chosen a way to monitor your progress toward that goal? If so, you are almost ready to start your 3-2-1 journey! In the next chapter, you will find some essential information that will help you to pick the best 3-2-1 meal plan and fitness plan for you.

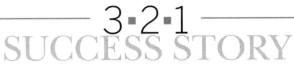

Anita Singh

Age: 30
Accomplishment: Lost 7 pounds and one dress size in five weeks

Q: How did you gain the excess weight?

A: I have been under a lot of stress recently. I changed jobs, planned my wedding, and took care of my husband through a liver illness. *Half* of the weight came from my honeymoon—I ate way too much, apparently.

Q: How does this weight loss plan compare to others you've tried?

A: I tried the South Beach Diet in the past with limited success. I also tried the Rice Diet—that system didn't work at all for me, and it was awful when I went out to eat. The last thing I tried was monitoring what I ate and exercising vigorously five or six times a week, but I didn't lose anything; I actually gained 5 pounds. So I decided I needed some guidance.

Q: What changes have you noticed in your physical health?

A: I am much more energetic, I am able to sleep more easily, and I know when I am full and when I'm hungry. I am amazed at the weight loss. I truly like knowing what I am putting into my system calorie-wise, and eating six times a day makes me feel full and satisfied.

Q: What changes have you noticed in your psychological health?

A: I feel very much in control of what I eat, and I haven't had the winter blues that I normally get this time of year. I've also noticed that I'm not as sensitive—things don't get me down as easily as they did before.

Q: How do your hunger and cravings fare on this plan compared to others you've tried?

A: On this plan, I haven't felt hungry or deprived, probably because of the treat I get to have at the end of the day. In fact, on some days, I felt too full to finish my meals! This is the opposite of how I felt on the South Beach Diet. During the first two weeks on that program, I felt sick, and I couldn't exercise because I had no energy. And boy, talk about feeling deprived! I always started to have a really hard time with it at Phase II and would have to start over again.

Q: What do you think of 3-2-1 exercise?

A: I love the exercise! It really gets me moving, and it's fun! On some days, at the beginning of the routine, I would fear that I wouldn't be able to make it through the whole session. Then all of a sudden, I was on the last circuit. That was a great feeling.

Q: What do you think of the food?

A: The food was very tasty and easy to prepare. I've been eating mostly frozen meals for lunch because they are the most convenient option. But I've been preparing the meals for dinner, and my husband really enjoys them. The 3-2-1 meal plan has been very easy to incorporate into my life, and I believe it has played the biggest role in my weight loss. The daily treat has been particularly instrumental in my success because it gives me something to eat other than fruits and veggies.

Q: Overall, what is your experience with 3-2-1?

A: Overall, my experience has been very positive. The 3-2-1 program is a whole lifestyle change—one that I am going to continue for life. The program has made me more active and has just been great for me overall. It's still amazing to me that I've lost 7 pounds in only a little over a month, especially with Thanksgiving being thrown in there! Thank you!

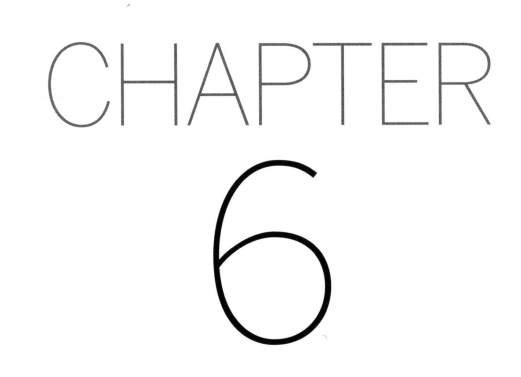

CHAPTER

6

PICK YOUR PLAN

HOW TO CUSTOMIZE THE PLAN
FOR YOUR BODY AND YOUR LIFE

In the coming chapters, you will find a three-phase program that will show you how to lose all the weight you want and then how to keep it off.

Phase 1 lasts one week. In this phase, you will ease into 3-2-1 exercise while you jump-start your weight loss with 3-2-1 eating. You'll see results by the end of this one-week phase, which will boost your motivation for Phase 2.

Phase 2 lasts until you lose all the weight you want. If you have only a little to lose, you might finish Phase 2 in just a few weeks. If you have 30 or more pounds to lose, it might take you months, or even a year.

Phase 3 is your maintenance phase. In those chapters, you'll learn how to modify your Phase 2 eating and fitness plans for long-term success.

For each phase of the plan, you'll find a suggested exercise routine along with meal plans of differing calorie levels. For best results, you'll need to modify each exercise routine (along with the suggested level of intensity and frequency) to your personal fitness level. You'll also need to choose the right meal plan to follow. You'll find out how to do both in the following pages.

PICK YOUR 3-2-1 FITNESS LEVEL

In this book, you'll find two 3-2-1 routines. The Phase 2 routine is a ramped-up version of the Phase 1 routine. If you are fit, you may already be ready for the Phase 2 routine. If you are out of shape, you may need to stick with the Phase 1 routine for longer than one week. To decide which routine to use and for how long, answer the following question.

How much do you currently exercise?

a. I've never exercised.

b. I used to exercise regularly but haven't done so in a few months.

c. I exercise fewer than three days a week but at least once a month.

d. I've been exercising for about a half hour three times a week for a few months or longer.

e. I exercise for 45 minutes or longer most days of the week.

If you answered (e) and you have less than 20 pounds to lose: Try the Phase 1 routine once to see how it feels. If it feels too easy, you can then progress to the Phase 2 routine, even as you follow the Phase 1 meal plan. Do not decrease your total exercise time. Your 3-2-1 routine will take you roughly 30 minutes to complete. If you currently exercise for longer, add extra cardio of your choice or do additional 3-2-1 circuits. For example, if you want to give your legs some extra attention, follow the 3-2-1 routine as prescribed, but then add an extra Legs and Shoulders Circuit and an extra Buns Circuit. If you are really fit, do the entire routine twice, for a total of 60 minutes.

If you answered (d) or (e): You'll probably do best if you start at the Phase 1 level. After one week, assess how you feel. If the routine felt relatively easy, then go directly to Phase 2. If parts of the routine felt very challenging, stick with the Phase 1 versions of those particular exercises, but otherwise move on to the Phase 2 routine. For example, you might do the Phase 2 strength-training moves with the Phase 1 cardio moves. If the entire routine felt very challenging, stick with the Phase 1 routine until you feel more comfortable and only then move on to Phase 2 exercise.

If you answered (b) or (c): You may be able to start with the full Phase 1 routine, but listen to your body. If you find that you must push yourself far beyond your comfort level (example: You wake the morning after your first try and are so sore you can barely get out of bed), start with half of the routine and work out every other day. For example, after a warmup on Monday, you would do the Arms, Legs and Shoulders, and Chest circuits. On Wednesday, the Buns and Back circuits. Then on Friday, the Arms, Legs and Shoulders, and Chest circuits again. Always pay attention to how you feel and take rest breaks between circuits as needed.

After a few weeks, try the entire routine, taking longer breaks between circuits and doing less than the recommended time if needed. Once you can do the entire routine in the prescribed time without rest breaks, you are officially in Phase 1. Stay in Phase 1 for at least one week before attempting any of the more advanced Phase 2 variations.

If you answered (a) and/or you have more than 20 pounds to lose: Try just one circuit at a time. For example, on Monday, do the Arms Circuit. On Tuesday, do the Buns Circuit. On Wednesday, do the Back Circuit. On Thursday, do the Legs and Shoulders Circuit. On Friday, do the Chest Circuit. This will give you 6 minutes of exercise a day (plus a few minutes of marching during your warmup and some stretching in your cooldown). After a few weeks—as you feel ready—double up your circuits, giving yourself a day of rest between sessions. For example, on Monday, do the Arms and Legs and Shoulders circuits. On Wednesday, do the Chest and Back circuits. On Friday, do the Legs and Shoulders and Buns circuits and repeat your favorite circuit.

Once that feels comfortable, do up to half of the 3-2-1 routine every other day. For example, after a warmup on Monday, you would do the Arms, Legs and Shoulders, and Chest circuits. On Wednesday, do the Buns and Back circuits. Then on Friday, do the Arms, Legs and Shoulders, and Chest circuits again. Take rest breaks between circuits as needed.

After a few weeks, try the entire routine. Take longer breaks between circuits and do fewer than the recommended number of reps if needed. Once you can do the entire routine at the prescribed number of reps without rest breaks, you are officially in Phase 1. Stay in Phase 1 for at least one week before attempting any of the more advanced Phase 2 variations.

PICK YOUR 3-2-1 MEAL PLAN

The 3-2-1 meal plans include three calorie levels: 1,200 calories, 1,500 calories, and 1,800 calories. In the following pages, you'll find guidelines for picking the right number of calories for your personal goal. Know that these guidelines are just that—guidelines. If, based on what you read in the following pages, you choose the 1,200 plan, but each day you feel ravenous, or shaky and lightheaded, you need more food and should move up to the 1,500 plan. Similarly, if you choose the 1,800 plan but just can't seem to lose any weight, you probably need to step down to 1,500.

The vast majority of the dieters I counsel do best on a 1,500-calorie plan. Nearly all women lose weight with that level of calories. However, if you are currently very overweight, you may be able to lose weight eating more. That's because the larger you are, the more calories your body naturally burns. On the other hand, if you have just a couple of pounds to lose, you'll probably need to eat less (smaller women burn fewer calories and typically require a lower-calorie plan in order to lose efficiently).

The Right Meal Plan for You

Consider the following factors when choosing your plan. Of course, people often fall into a number of categories, so be sure to listen to your body. If you feel ravenously hungry as you start the plan, you should try the next higher calorie level. On the other hand, if you're following the plan closely and you're not seeing results, revise your calorie goals down to the next lower level. Use this chart to help determine the best plan for you, then read on for more information about each factor listed.

1,200-Calorie Plan

Small-framed women

Short women (5' 2" or less)

Women over age 40

Postmenopausal women

Sedentary women (inactive with moderate planned exercise three times a week or less)

1,500-Calorie Plan

Medium-framed women

Women of average height (5' 2" to 5' 6")

Women under age 40

Premenopausal women

Women who exercise moderately (up to 30 minutes five days a week)

1,800-Calorie Plan

Large-framed women

Women with more than 30 pounds to lose

Tall women (5' 6" or taller)

Women who exercise vigorously (more than 45 minutes five days a week)

Exercise level: Exercise burns calories. The more you exercise, the more you can eat and still lose weight. The less you exercise, the less you can eat. The 3-2-1 plan recommends you exercise for 30 minutes three times a week during Phase 1 and four times a week during Phase 2. If you are sedentary, you will start with less exercise, and if you are very fit, you might start with more (see page 117 to pick the right level for you). If you are starting with just 6 daily minutes of exercise, you may do very well on the 1,200-calorie plan. Once you move up to the recommended amount of exercise (30 minutes three times a week), you will need to move up to the 1,500-calorie plan. Similarly, if you're already exercising a lot—45 to 60 minutes a day—you'll probably be able to lose weight on the 1,800-calorie plan (and will need that number of calories to avoid intense hunger).

Age: Metabolism usually slows with age and takes a dip at menopause, so the older you are, the fewer calories you can eat without gaining weight. If you are older than 40 or postmenopausal, the 1,200-calorie plan may work best for you, especially if you are currently sedentary.

Amount of weight you want to lose: If you have 30 or more pounds to lose, the 1,800-calorie plan probably makes the most sense for you (unless you're menopausal or post-menopausal, in which case you may want to choose the 1,500-calorie plan). On the other hand, if you only have 5 or 10 pounds to lose, go ahead and follow the 1,200-calorie plan for a couple of weeks to reach your goal quickly. Then move straight to Phase 3.

Height: If you are tall, you burn more calories than a shorter woman. If you are at least 5' 6", you may be able to lose weight on the 1,800-calorie plan, especially if you exercise at least three times a week. If you're less than 5' 2", you may need the 1,200-calorie plan to lose weight.

The Best Plan for You Over Time

The best calorie level for you today may not continue to be the best level for you as you progress along the 3-2-1 program, for two reasons.

1. If you have more than 30 pounds to lose, you'll probably start with the 1,800-calorie plan. As you lose weight and your body becomes smaller, your basal metabolic rate (the rate at which your body burns calories to power your heartbeat and other essential functions) naturally goes down. This is one reason almost all dieters hit a plateau.

2. As you become more fit, you will burn more calories. You may start on the 1,200-calorie plan, but as you add more exercise minutes to your day, you may find that you are too hungry and require more food to fuel your body. Thus, you need to switch to a higher-calorie plan.

How do you know when it's time to eat less or eat more?

First, let's talk about eating less. If you start with the 1,800-calorie plan and lose weight consistently, but then hit a plateau that lasts longer than three weeks, it's probably time to switch to the 1,500-calorie plan. Before you switch, however, check to make sure your plateau is not caused by other factors (see Chapter 13). Make sure, for example, that you are following the 1,800-calorie plan as written and not including seemingly hidden sources of calories such as extra dressing on your salad, cream in your coffee, or butter on your bread. Similarly, check to make sure you are doing the right amount of exercise. If everything checks out, then it's time to make the switch.

Now let's talk about eating more. If, long after the first two weeks of dieting, you begin to lose more than 2 pounds a week, it's time to add more food to your plate. If you start to feel hungry most of the time, jittery, or lightheaded, consider that a good sign that you need more food. Allowing yourself to lose weight too quickly will leave you dehydrated and tired. Worse, rapid weight loss generally comes from muscle rather than fat, which slows your metabolism and makes it harder to reach your long-term goal. So eat more now. You'll benefit in the long run.

I know, I know, it feels odd to eat more and continue to lose weight. But it happens! I've counseled many dieters who were sedentary when they first came to me and who, truth be told, had no plans to exercise at all. One in particular, Margie, was working long hours at a desk as an executive assistant. She didn't have time to exercise and had no motivation to fit it in. So I started her on the 1,200-calorie plan. She lost 15 pounds on this plan and, as a result, felt more energetic. On the weekends, she began enjoying

3·2·1 SUCCESS STORY

Tina Cundiff

Age: 41
Major Accomplishment: Avoided large weight gain while quitting smoking—shrank 2 inches from her waist instead

Q: How did you gain the excess weight?
A: I ate way too many sweets, had a hysterectomy, and tried to quit smoking a few times, all of which contributed to my weight gain.

Q: Why did you choose to go on the 3-2-1 program?
A: This plan seemed right for me because I am not good at planning my meals or planning my exercise—I needed some guidance. Plus, I really, really needed to quit smoking. So I figured if I could give my metabolism a bit of a jump with the program, I wouldn't gain weight as I was trying to quit. In all my past attempts to quit, I have always put the pounds on. So I didn't go on the program so much to lose weight, but to avoid gaining weight as I was quitting smoking, and it worked!

Q: What changes have you noticed in your physical health?
A: My energy level is high, and I definitely feel stronger. It's easier for me to do my daily chores. More important, although I didn't lose weight on the scale, I lost 2" off my waist!

all sorts of fun physical activity. She played tennis outdoors, walked on the beach, and even ran around the playground with her kids. Eventually, she found that she *wanted* to exercise. So during the week, she'd get up on two or three mornings at 5:00 a.m. in order to fit in a workout. Then she'd shower, grab breakfast on her way out the door, and eat it on the train during her commute. The extra exercise meant that she could in no way continue to follow the 1,200-calorie plan, so we bumped her up to 1,500, and she continued to lose weight while eating more food.

3-2-1 GO!

Now that you've set your goal and chosen the right plan to follow, you are ready to lose. Turn to Chapter 7 to find out everything you need to know about Phase 1.

Q: What changes have you noticed in your psychological health?
A: Using the program in conjunction with quitting smoking has helped me successfully quit. I am more confident than ever before that this time I will remain a nonsmoker. Today, it has been 49 days since my last cigarette!

Q: How did your hunger and cravings fare on this plan compared to others you've tried?
A: I have no hunger on the food plan. In fact, it is just the opposite. It is actually too much food for me.

Q: What did you think about the exercise?
A: The exercise is wonderful. I look forward to doing the workout every other day, and I upped my hand weights from 5 to 10 pounds.

Q: Overall, what was your experience like with 3-2-1?
A: It has been great! I will continue with the exercise program and healthy eating. I don't see it as a weight loss plan, but as a total change in my way of living. Although I didn't lose weight, I only gained 2 pounds through quitting smoking, and I suspect some of that is due to the weight training on the program. All in all, I am very happy with my results! Thank you for the opportunity!

PART II

Phase 1

CHAPTER

7

ABOUT PHASE 1

WHAT YOU NEED TO KNOW BEFORE YOU START

Phase 1 of your 3-2-1 journey will last one week. During this short but effective phase of the 3-2-1 program you will ease into 3-2-1 exercise as you jump-start your weight loss with 3-2-1 eating. By the end of this week, you can expect to have lost up to 6 pounds.

In Chapter 8, you will find seven days' worth of menus for three different calorie levels: 1,200 calories, 1,500 calories, and 1,800 calories. Each of the calorie plans follows the same format. No matter whether you are following the 1,200 plan, the 1,500 plan, or the 1,800 plan, you will find whole grain cereal on the menu for breakfast for Day 1. Similarly, all plans call for salmon fillets with salsa for lunch on Day 5. The meal options for breakfast, lunch, and dinner are the same on most days (with a few exceptions here and there). The higher-calorie plans, however, include larger snacks and additional side dishes and larger portions at various meals.

In the Phase 1 meal plan, I've made your shift to 3-2-1 eating as easy and straightforward as possible. You'll find many quick and easy options that you can grab and eat on the run. You'll also find numerous omelets, salads, and sandwiches because those options are convenient and have repeatedly topped the "most favorite foods" lists of the thousands of clients I've counseled over the years. For the same reason, you'll also find yogurt with fruit, oatmeal, and a tomato-and-cheese melt. If you enjoy cooking more gourmet fare, then you'll love Salmon with Spicy Salsa and Chicken with White Wine and Mushrooms. I've included a little of everything. I'm confident that you'll find something that works for you.

For optimal success, feel free to modify the options to fit your personal tastes and lifestyle. I provide plenty of variety throughout the week and include suggestions in the plan for making a few specific substitutions. I don't expect you to love every single meal option, so don't get put off if you see meals that you don't want to cook or eat. Feel free to mix and match various breakfasts, lunches, and dinners. Repeat the turkey sandwich for lunch a few times. Go ahead and have the egg-white omelet again if you desire. All of the meals are interchangeable. You can even eat the same breakfast every day if that approach pleases you.

Here is specific advice to help you modify the meal plan for your personal tastes and lifestyle.

Go vegetarian if needed. You may substitute tofu or tempeh for meat, chicken, or fish. For tofu, double the amount listed for meat, chicken, or fish. For tempeh, the amount remains the same as what's listed. You may substitute veggie burgers for burgers made with beef or turkey meat.

Go lactose free if needed. You may substitute low-fat soy milk or fat-free Lactaid milk for the same amount of cow's milk listed on any given day. You also may use soy cheese or vegetable cheese in place of regular low-fat cheese. The same goes for soy yogurt.

Omit cheese as needed. Some people are cheese lovers; others are anything but. If you fall into the latter category, feel free to omit any cheese suggested for a meal, instead increasing your serving of lean protein in that meal by 1 to 2 ounces. For example, on the 1,800-calorie plan on Day 3, you will find a turkey and cheese sandwich. If you don't like cheese, omit it and add an additional slice or two of turkey.

Double—but don't triple—red meat. If you skim through the plan, you'll see that I include red meat only once (you can look forward to a juicy sirloin steak on Day 7). Although you can eat any other suggested dinner option as often as you want (for example, having the Day 1 dinner every day), Day 7 is an exception to that rule. From a nutritional standpoint, I recommend you eat red meat no more than twice a week. Red meat typically contains more calories than other leaner types of protein. Also, more frequent consumption of higher-fat red meat may increase your risk of certain cancers and other diseases. If you love red meat, go ahead and enjoy the Day 7 dinner twice during the week—but no more.

ABOUT PHASE 1 DINNERS

The Phase 1 dinner options do not include grains or starchy vegetables. I've completely omitted these carbohydrates with dinner for the first seven days in order to encourage you to fill up on low-calorie, high-fiber vegetables such as spinach, broccoli, cauliflower, asparagus, and others. Most dinner options come with a nonstarchy vegetable side dish, plus a large salad that often allows for an unlimited amount of lettuce, spinach, or other leafy greens.

This abundance of vegetables will help fill you up while keeping your calorie intake low. This strategy also helps prevent overeating at dinner—as well as afterward. Most people, when they overeat at dinner, do so by eating too much potato, rice, pasta, or other grain or starch. By omitting this problematic meal component for one week, you will better be able to train yourself to first fill up on vegetables before going overboard on grains. If you are the type of person who needs volume to feel satisfied after eating, then pile on the lettuce and other unlimited greens. Use these super low calorie vegetables to satisfy your urge to chew as well as to satisfy your hunger.

Not only do these low-calorie vegetables fill you up, they are also great for your health. The carrots, peppers, dark leafy greens, brussels sprouts, asparagus, and other vegetable offerings are loaded with vitamins, minerals, fiber, and health-promoting phytochemicals that reduce the risk of cancer, heart disease, and other physical ailments.

Although the meal plans recommend specific amounts of certain vegetables, this is the place where you can relax your portion-control standards. While you absolutely must eat the correct portions of meat, grains, condiments, salad dressings, and other foods, you have much more room for error when it comes to nonstarchy vegetables. If the menu calls for 8 asparagus spears but you eat 14, don't sweat it. Relax. These vegetables are all so low in calories that a few extra will not greatly affect your calorie bottom line.

What if you see a vegetable that you don't like? Feel free to substitute another vegetable that you do like. You can substitute any of the following vegetables for the same amount of any nonstarchy vegetable: asparagus, beets, broccoli, brussels sprouts, cabbage, carrots, cauliflower, celery, cucumbers, eggplant, green beans, greens (collard, mustard, and turnip), kale, kohlrabi, leeks, lettuce, mushrooms, okra, onions, pea pods, peppers (red, yellow, and green), radishes, rutabaga, spinach, Swiss chard, tomatoes, water chestnuts, and zucchini.

HOW TO EAT OUT ON THE PLAN

I understand it's unrealistic to eat all meals at home, every single day. Restaurants are part of most of our lives—both for convenience and social pleasure. That said, here's how to stick with your 3-2-1 plan and still enjoy an occasional outing.

To follow the Phase 1 meal plan at your favorite restaurants, simply order a restaurant meal similar to any meal you find on the plan. You probably won't be able to order exactly what is prescribed, but you can get close. Watch portion sizes closely, especially the portions for meats and fats (such as salad dressings and margarine).

Calories can add up quickly in restaurants, which typically serve portions double or triple what you should eat to lose weight. You may need to halve your portions as soon as your food comes to the table, putting half of the meal in a takeout container. (Because the 3-2-1 meals are interchangeable, you can enjoy the leftovers the next day.)

To watch your portions, learn to pay attention to the sizes of your meals at home when you have control over food preparation. That will help you to learn what proper portions look like for when you eat out. Also use the following visual rules of thumb.

Meat: 1 ounce is the size of a matchbox. 3 ounces is the size of a deck of cards.

Fish: 3 ounces is the size of a checkbook.

Cheese: 1 ounce is the size of four dice.

Pasta, rice, and other grains: ½ cup is the size of half a tennis ball.

Breakfast

These breakfast choices, modified from the Phase 1 meal plans, will keep you on track when dining out.

Egg-white omelet: Most breakfast establishments serve egg whites or egg substitute these days. Get an egg-white omelet with any vegetable combination you like (peppers, onions, tomatoes, etc.). The restaurant probably won't have whole wheat pitas, so substitute one slice of whole wheat toast without butter, margarine, or jelly.

Oatmeal: Any breakfast place will serve you a bowl of oatmeal. Ask for fat-free milk on the side and top the oatmeal with sliced strawberries. Skip the sugar—use sugar substitute if you prefer your oatmeal to be sweetened.

Vegetable omelet: This meal is similar to the egg-white omelet. In the meal plan, the vegetable omelet calls for fat-free cheese, which your restaurant probably will not offer. Order an egg-white omelet with any vegetables you desire and ask the wait staff to go very light on the cheese. If you are following one of the plans that calls for fruit, order the same amount of any fruit the restaurant offers.

Lunch

Here are good options for eating lunch out, taken from the Phase 1 meal plan.

Turkey burger: If the restaurant doesn't offer a turkey burger, check for other options, such as a veggie burger. If nothing is available but beef, then go ahead and have a beef burger. The restaurant probably will not have black bean salad, so instead, if you are on the 1,200-calorie plan, enjoy your burger on half a bun with a side salad tossed with fresh lemon juice and/or balsamic vinegar; don't add salad dressing. If you are following the 1,500-calorie plan, eat the whole bun and follow the same salad rules as for the 1,200-calorie plan. If you're on the 1,800-calorie plan, enjoy the whole bun and toss your side salad with 1 tablespoon regular dressing or 2 tablespoons low-calorie dressing.

Turkey sandwich: You can get a turkey sandwich from just about any deli for lunch. But you probably won't find reduced-calorie bread, so order your sandwich on whole wheat toast and remove the top slice, eating the sandwich open faced (if you're following the 1,800-calorie plan, you can enjoy both slices of regular bread). Use mustard instead of mayo and order either baby carrots or pickles on the side. Decline the potato chips that will probably come with the meal.

Cottage cheese with fresh fruit: Make sure the cottage cheese is low fat. Forgo the wheat germ suggested in the meal plan if the restaurant doesn't have it. Order whatever fruit the restaurant offers, keeping the portions equal to what's described in your plan.

Dinner

Here are smart options for dinner, modified for restaurant eating from the Phase 1 meal plan.

Chicken teriyaki with vegetables: You will find this meal at most Asian restaurants. Make sure the vegetables are steamed, not fried, and not covered in sauce. Use extra sauce from your chicken to flavor the steamed vegetables. Decline the rice that will probably come with the meal. If you are following one of the meal plans that calls for fruit with this dish, enjoy any fruit that the restaurant offers, keeping the portions equal.

Grilled chicken Caesar salad: Most restaurants serve a grilled chicken Caesar salad. When you order, ask to have it *without* the dressing or croutons. For dressing, you can request Caesar on the side and use only 1 tablespoon, ask for low-calorie dressing on the side and enjoy 2 to 4 tablespoons, or request oil and vinegar on the side and use up to 1 teaspoon olive oil and as much vinegar as you want.

Grilled salmon: Most restaurants serve this standard dish. Feel free to swap the salmon for any other grilled, roasted, or baked fish. Order the fish with whatever steamed vegetables the restaurant offers; ask to double the serving of plain vegetables and hold

3•2•1 **TIP** No need to take measuring spoons with you to the restaurant to measure your salad dressing. At home, measure out the right amount of dressing a few times so you can see how many shakes to give yourself when eating out.

the rice, potatoes, or other starch that may come with your meal. If you'd like to spice up this dish, ask for a side of salsa or hot sauce and spoon it over your fish at the table.

Grilled sirloin: You can find sirloin at any steak house, but it will probably come in a much larger portion than you should eat. Before heading to the restaurant, make sure you know what a 4-ounce serving (if you are on the 1,200-calorie plan) or a 6-ounce serving (if you are on the 1,500 or 1,800 plan) looks like. Three ounces of steak is roughly the size of a deck of cards. Four is slightly more than that, and 6 ounces is the size of two card decks. Your steak will probably be 12 ounces, so cut away one-half or two-thirds of the steak as soon as it gets to the table and put it in a take-home container. Instead of the tomato and mozzarella salad (which steak restaurants typically don't have), order plain tomato and onion slices and drizzle with plain balsamic vinegar—not balsamic vinaigrette. Order spinach or another vegetable in place of whatever starch (rice, baked potato, or pasta) would normally come with the meal.

3-2-1 EMERGENCY OPTIONS

When designing the meals you'll find in Phase 1, I have tried to choose options that require as little preparation as possible. That said, I know there will be days when any amount of chopping just may not cut it for you. On those days, you can still follow 3-2-1 and lose weight. Consider these options.

Keep a stash of frozen dinners on hand. While I don't recommend you eat frozen dinners every day (many contain more sodium than you need), they do provide a nice option on busy days. In this phase of the plan, you will not be eating high-quality starch (brown rice, quinoa, whole wheat pasta, baked potato) with dinner, so look for dinner entrées that do not incorporate starchy vegetables or grains. If you choose a dinner that does have a grain or starch, put it aside and instead enjoy either fresh fruit (consult the meal plans for types and serving sizes), additional plain vegetables (steamed or microwaved fresh or frozen veggies), or a side salad of prewashed, prechopped salad mix and 2 to 4 tablespoons low-calorie salad dressing.

Here is a guide for choosing frozen dinners based on the calorie breakdown for your plan.

- **1,200-calorie plan:** Choose any entrée with 350 calories or less
- **1,500-calorie plan:** Choose any entrée with 400 calories or less. Serve with 1 cup baby carrots or half a grapefruit.

- **1,800-calorie plan:** Choose any entrée with 400 calories with less. Serve with 1 cup baby carrots *and* an unlimited amount of steamed, boiled, or microwaved vegetables (such as cauliflower, green beans, spinach, or broccoli) topped with 4 tablespoons Parmesan cheese.

Keep ingredients for this 3-minute meal (1,200-calorie plan) on hand. Place as much as an entire bag of prewashed leafy greens on a dinner plate. Drain a 5-ounce can of light tuna (packed in water), chicken breast, or wild salmon and place on the greens. Toss with 2 to 4 tablespoons low-calorie dressing of your choice.

If you are following the 1,500-calorie plan: Add 1 ounce crumbled feta cheese or 1 ounce grated reduced-fat hard cheese.

If you are following the 1,800-calorie plan: Add 2 tablespoons chopped nuts or seeds (any type) or have just 1 tablespoon of nuts and enjoy half a grapefruit on the side.

CALORIE BREAKDOWNS BY PLAN

Below you will find the calorie breakdowns for each plan. Understanding your breakdown can help when certain foods are not available or practical. Use these breakdowns to choose frozen dinners or alter 3-2-1 meals to fit your personal tastes.

1,200-Calorie Plan

Breakfast: 200 calories	**Lunch:** 300 calories	**Dinner:** 350 calories
AM Snack: 100 calories	**PM Snack:** 100 calories	**Treat:** 150 calories

1,500-Calorie Plan

Breakfast: 250 calories	**Lunch:** 400 calories	**Dinner:** 450 calories
AM Snack: 100 calories	**PM Snack:** 150 calories	**Treat:** 150 calories

1,800-Calorie Plan

Breakfast: 300 calories	**Lunch:** 450 calories	**Dinner:** 550 calories
AM Snack: 150 calories	**PM Snack:** 200 calories	**Treat:** 150 calories

A WORD ABOUT YOUR SNACKS

If you take a moment to skim the meal plans, you'll see that you can choose a morning and afternoon snack (you'll find Snack Lists on pages 320–25). Although the plan suggests you eat one snack in the morning and one in the afternoon, you may alter the timing as needed.

For example, if you are the type of person who rises early, fits in a workout, and eats breakfast by 7:00 a.m. but doesn't eat lunch until 1:00 p.m., you'll absolutely need that morning snack. On the other hand, if you are a late riser who eats breakfast during your commute to work and then has an early lunch, you may not need the morning snack at all. In that case, you might take the 100 calories from your morning snack and use them to beef up the portion of your protein at lunch or dinner by 2 ounces (the size of two matchboxes).

Similarly, if you tend to feel hungry by midafternoon and suffer from afternoon slump, that's a great time for your afternoon snack. On the other hand, if you tend to need to eat a little something to avoid overeating at dinner, have your snack during your commute home from the office or as you prepare your dinner. Finally, if you are the type of person who likes to eat at night, you might even save your afternoon snack until after dinner.

There are no hard-and-fast rules—*as long as* you eat every 4 to 5 hours and *as long as* you follow an eating pattern that works for your personal hunger and lifestyle. You can put your snacks where you want them, but try to follow the same pattern each day. Get in a rhythm. You follow a set rhythm for work, arriving at the same time and leaving around the same time each day. You probably follow a rhythm in your television habits, watching the same shows at the same times. Do the same with your eating. Your rhythm will help make 3-2-1 more habitual, so you will eat every four to five hours without thinking about it, just as you brush your teeth before bed each night without thinking about it.

A WORD ABOUT YOUR TREATS

On 3-2-1, you have the option of eating a treat from the Phase 1 Treat List (page 314) every day. Keep in mind that you don't have to eat your treat if you don't need or want it. If you don't feel a craving for something sweet or fun, but you are still hungry, you can skip the treat and instead have an extra serving of fruit or starch or an additional 2 ounces of protein. To make the swap, use these serving sizes.

One serving of fruit equals

1 medium apple	1 nectarine
½ cup unsweetened applesauce	1 orange
4 apricots	1 peach
1 cup berries	1 medium pear
¼ cantaloupe or 1 cup cubed melon	2 persimmons
12 large cherries	1 cup pineapple
2 clementines	½ pomegranate
2 figs	2 small plums
½ grapefruit	2 tablespoons raisins
20 grapes	1½ cups whole strawberries
1 kiwi	2 tangerines
½ mango	1 medium watermelon wedge

One serving of starch equals

½ cup acorn or butternut squash	½ cup corn
2 slices reduced-calorie bread	½ whole grain English muffin
1 slice whole wheat bread	½ cup kidney beans
½ regular whole wheat pita bread	½ cup dry plain oatmeal
1 small whole wheat pita bread (70 calories)	½ cup cooked whole wheat pasta
¾ cup whole grain breakfast cereal (120 calories or less)	½ cup peas
	½ medium baked white potato
½ cup chickpeas	½ medium baked sweet potato
	½ cup cooked brown or wild rice

If you are not in the mood for your treat and you don't feel hungry, just skip it. You'll save yourself 150 calories. Know, however, that your treat is always there for you. Don't *try* to skip the treat. You can and should have your treat when you need it. Remember: Deprivation leads to overeating.

In Phase 1, all of the treats on your list are indulgent yet healthy. Whether you choose red wine, dark chocolate, or pudding, they all contain health-promoting phytonutrients, vitamins, or minerals along with delicious taste satisfaction.

Eat your treat when you crave it most. For the majority of people I counsel, this means having it at night. Doing so gives you something to look forward to all day long, helping you to eat the right foods in the right portions at lunch and dinner.

Some people do best, in fact, if they eat their treats right before bed. If you are one of them, you know who you are. If you are reading this and can't imagine eating before bed, then don't. It's that simple.

But don't worry about calories turning into fat as you sleep. This just isn't true. I know this from working with thousands and thousands of clients who ate their treats at night and did not get fatter by morning! If eating your treat before bed prevents you from overeating all night long, you will definitely lose weight. If eating before bed gives you indigestion or disturbs your sleep, however, a before-bed treat just isn't right for you.

You may choose any treat from the Treat List as long as:

• You eat the treat in the prescribed portion.

• You stay away from your trigger foods, the ones that cause you to lose control and don't allow you to hold yourself to a portion-controlled serving.

A WORD ABOUT SUPPLEMENTS

I don't recommend weight loss supplements. The 3-2-1 meal plan and exercise plan are all you need to lose weight, so there's no need to spend extra money on fat burners or appetite suppressants you see in health food stores.

That said, to help fill in any nutritional gaps, I strongly recommend that you consider taking a multivitamin-mineral supplement as well as a separate daily calcium supplement with vitamin D (especially if you're a woman who doesn't eat enough dairy foods).

Please note: If you have any preexisting medical concerns, always speak with your physician before taking any new supplements.

How to Choose a Multivitamin

Your multi should contain roughly 100 percent of the Daily Value (DV) for *most* vitamins and minerals. The minerals calcium and magnesium are exceptions, however, as 100 percent of the DV for these minerals simply will not fit into a multivitamin that you can actually swallow (which is one reason why I recommend you take your calcium separately). If you can, try to find a multivitamin that contains at least 50 percent of the DV for magnesium.

Here are a few additional hints for choosing a multivitamin.

• Few multivitamins contain 100 percent of the DV for vitamin K. Look for at least 25 micrograms of K if you are premenopausal and 10 micrograms if you are older than age 50. This vitamin can interfere with blood thinners; if you are taking Coumadin (warfarin) or another blood thinner, speak with your doctor before taking a multi with K.

• Avoid supplements that feature high amounts of vitamin A in the form of retinol or palmitate. Too much straight vitamin A can raise the risk of hip fractures, liver disease, and birth defects. Ideally, your supplement should contain no more than 2,000 IU of vitamin A from palmitate or retinol, and the rest should come from mixed carotenoids or beta-carotene. These forms are safe, and the body converts them into vitamin A as needed.

• If you are older than age 50, look for a formula that does *not* contain iron. Too much iron may suppress the immune system, and many multivitamins contain much more of this mineral than many people need. If you are pre-menopausal, choose one that contains no more than 18 milligrams of iron.

How to Choose a Calcium Supplement

Adequate consumption of calcium helps to prevent osteoporosis, the demineralizing and weakening of bones. If you're younger than age 50, you need 1,000 milligrams of calcium a day. If you're older than 50, you need 1,200 milligrams. To consume this amount in food, you would need to eat three to four servings of a calcium-rich food every day, which can be difficult when you are losing weight—especially if you are following the 1,200-calorie plan. Taking a supplement provides insurance and protection on those days when your consumption may be low.

Use these tips to pick the right supplement for you.

• Purchase either calcium carbonate or citrate. Calcium carbonate must be taken with food.

• Take 500 to 600 milligrams of calcium twice a day, for a total of 1,000 to 1,200 milligrams.

• Look for a supplement that contains vitamin D_3 (or cholecalciferol, the most bioactive type of vitamin D). It enhances the absorption of calcium into the bone. You need it not only for strong bones but also to reduce the risk of certain cancers and autoimmune diseases. Ideally, you want about 400 IU of D from your multivitamin and another 200 to 400 from calcium supplements.

3·2·1
SUCCESS STORY

Lori Wilson

Age: 44

Accomplishment: Lost 10 pounds in three weeks and dropped two dress sizes (16 to 14)

Q: How did you gain the excess weight?

A: I gained most of my excess 40 pounds when I was in an unhappy relationship. I have since ended that relationship and am pursuing another one. This is part of the reason I have renewed my efforts to lose weight. Of course, he told me he loves me no matter what I look like, but I told him that I don't.

Q: How does this weight loss plan compare to others you've tried?

A: I think I've tried every other diet on the face of the earth and nothing has really compared to this one. I've tried numerous diet plans and diet aids—Dexatrim, Hydroxycut, and Weight Watchers, to name a few. Most important, the 3-2-1 weight loss plan is convenient. The meals are easy to prepare, and I like that I can eat real food rather than always having "prepared frozen meals." I've never had cravings, with the exception of a certain time of the month. I am totally satisfied with what I am able to eat. I don't use the treat often because I don't feel as if I need it! I am always full and satisfied. For all the other diets I've tried, I struggled to motivate myself to exercise beyond walking. The results I achieved plus the energy I feel on this plan help me find the motivation to exercise.

Q: What changes have you noticed in your psychological health?

A: I have more energy to exercise, which was something that I didn't to do before. My mood has changed tremendously due to the weight loss and ability to wear smaller-size clothes. It has motivated me even more to reach the goal I have set for myself. My boyfriend has noticed the change, as have my coworkers.

Q: Would you recommend this program to a friend?

A: I enjoy this plan more than any I have tried. It does not feel like a diet to me but rather a change in my life—a good change. I salute anyone who does this weight loss plan. Try it, and, believe me, you will succeed.

LADIES, START YOUR 3-2-1 JOURNEY

Now you know everything you need to successfully follow the first week of 3-2-1 nutrition and exercise. I'm confident that you will love this new way of eating and moving your body. Once you start eating every 4 to 5 hours and doing the 3-2-1 circuits, you'll never again want to return to your old ways. So get started. Turn to Chapter 8 to find your first week of menus and your exercise routine at a glance. Plan what you will eat. Stock your kitchen with the ingredients you need and start eating and exercising your way to a slimmer, healthier body!

CHAPTER 8

PHASE 1

WHAT TO DO EACH DAY

In the following pages, you will find seven days' worth of meal suggestions along with small photos that show your Phase 1 exercise routine at a glance. You have everything you need here to see dramatic results in just seven days.

Use these pointers when following your meal plan.

Beware of adding extracurricular calories. On this meal plan, I've accounted for every last calorie, down to the salad dressing and mustard. Feel free to modify the plan to fit your needs, but try not to add condiments and other flavorings in amounts above what the plan recommends. If the menu calls for reduced-fat mayo, don't use regular mayo instead. If it calls for a packet of sugar, you may *omit* the sugar or use a sugar substitute, but don't add *two* packs of sugar. It may be a good idea, in fact, to measure out salad dressing, condiments, sour cream, and other additions in the beginning, until you can get a feel for what proper portions look like. And be sure to use a teaspoon (not a tablespoon) when instructed—since there are 3 teaspoons in 1 tablespoon, it makes a big difference (especially for calorie-dense items like olive oil, peanut butter, and margarine spreads).

Avoid liquid calories. You may drink unlimited amounts of water, seltzer, plain coffee, tea, and other calorie-free beverages. but avoid adding calories to these drinks by putting cream in your coffee or honey in your tea, for example. If you are caffeine sensitive, choose decaffeinated versions or limit your coffee and tea consumption, opting for water instead.

You may use artificial sweeteners. Diet beverages and other artificially sweetened foods will not impede your weight loss in any way, but if you choose to include these items, please do so in moderation (no more than one or two artificially sweetened items each day).

Feel free to kick things up a notch. You may use unlimited amounts of the following seasonings: basil, bay leaves, celery seed, chili powder, chives, cinnamon, cumin, curry, dill, flavoring extracts (such as almond and vanilla), garlic powder, hot pepper sauce, lemon, lemon juice, lemon pepper, lime juice, minced onion, onion powder, oregano, paprika, parsley, pepper, pimiento, low-sodium soy sauce, tarragon, thyme, turmeric, and vinegar.

If you eat more than the plan calls for at a given meal, get right back on track. Whether you go off the plan completely or have just a few extra spoonfuls, do not give up for the entire day, week, or month. Get back on track at the very next meal or snack. If possible, try to undo the overeating by taking an extra walk or skipping your treat.

YOUR 3-2-1 PROGRESS REPORT

Before you start, I'd like you to take a moment to fill in your first 3-2-1 Progress Report. As I mentioned in Chapter 5, monitoring your success only by the scale can backfire. To stay motivated even when you hit a plateau, I'd like you to rate the following on a scale of 0 to 10 (with 0 indicating the worst you've ever felt and 10 indicating the most fantastic you ever could feel).

How you feel about your health .... ☐

How you feel about your level of energy .... ☐

How you feel about your weight and body .... ☐

How you feel about your level of commitment to losing weight .... ☐

You will complete a new 3-2-1 Progress Report each week during the first month of your 3-2-1 weight loss journey. After that, you will do so once a month until you reach your goal. Write down your ratings in a notebook so you can compare notes from week to week to see if you are moving in the right direction.

As you progress along 3-2-1, you can expect your level of commitment to wax and wane. After a while, the newness of 3-2-1 will wear off. Some days will feel harder than others, some easier than others. If any given rating of your level of commitment falls below a 5, reread Chapter 4 to help find ways to motivate yourself to move forward. Also focus on the improvements in your other ratings. You will notice, if you compare ratings, that you'll most definitely feel better about your weight, energy, and health as your journey unfolds.

YOUR PHASE 1 GROCERY LIST

I want you to feel free to mix and match your meals. To make things easier on you, I have created a grocery list. It contains all of the food items you will probably need during the first week of 3-2-1—and beyond. It includes everything you would need if you followed the 3-2-1 menus and recipes day by day without fail. This list is based on the 1,200-calorie plan and includes specific advice for the 1,500 and 1,800 plans as well. It also includes some staples that appear often in the 3-2-1 recipes as well as suggestions for foods you should consider stocking in your freezer today—in case you have unexpected conflicts tomorrow and don't have the time to prepare the 3-2-1 lunch or dinner that you planned. If you take the time to stock up on these ingredients now, you'll need to shop for only the fresh items (skinless chicken breast, wild salmon, and fresh vegetables and fruit) as you need them.

Condiments, Spices, and Oils

Keep the following items on hand, replacing them as you use them up.

Allspice, ground

Cinnamon, ground

Cooking spray

Cumin, ground

Hot pepper sauce

Maple syrup, lite (reduced-sugar)

Mayonnaise, reduced-fat

Mustard, Dijon or yellow

Mustard, onion-flavored

Nutmeg

Oil, canola

Oil, olive

Oregano, dried

Pepper, black

Pepper, red (cayenne)

Pepper, white

Rosemary, dried

Sage, dried

Salt or salt substitute

Soy sauce, low-sodium (or low-sodium teriyaki sauce)

Tabasco sauce (optional)

Thyme, dried

Vanilla extract

Vinegar

Vinegar, balsamic

Dry/Canned Goods

After opening, refrigerate the items that require it, such as dressings, applesauce, and mayonnaise.

Applesauce, natural

Baking powder

Beans, black, canned

Bread, whole grain, reduced-calorie (45 calories or less per slice)

Broth, chicken, reduced-fat

Buns, hamburger, whole grain (120 calories or less per bun)

Cereal, whole grain (120 calories or less and 3 or more grams of fiber per ¾ to 1 cup)

Chickpeas, canned

Corn, canned

Cornstarch

Dressing, Caesar, low-calorie (80 calories or less per 2 tablespoons)

Dressing, salad, low-calorie or fat-free (40 calories or less per 2 tablespoons)

Flour, all-purpose

Oatmeal (dry traditional oatmeal or quick-cooking oats)

Peanut butter, preferably natural (or almond or soy nut butter)

Pitas, mini, whole wheat (70 calories or less per pita)

Salmon, wild, canned

Salsa (20 calories or less per 2 tablespoons)

Sugar, brown

Sugar, granulated

Sugar substitute

Tahini (sesame paste)

Tuna, light, canned, packed in water

Walnuts (or pecans or slivered almonds)

Wheat bran

Wheat germ

1,500- and 1,800-Calorie Plans Only

1,500-calorie plan: Omit bread listed above and use reduced-calorie whole grain bread (80 calories or less per slice) instead.

1,800-calorie plan: Omit bread listed above and instead use reduced-calorie whole grain bread (120 calories or less per slice).

Dairy and Eggs

Keep the following on hand at all times.

Cheese, American, reduced-fat

Cheese, mozzarella, part-skim

Cheese, Parmesan

Cottage cheese, fat-free or
  1% reduced-fat

Eggs

Egg whites or egg substitute

Margarine spread, reduced-fat, soft tub,
  trans fat–free

Milk, fat-free or 1%

Yogurt, fat-free, vanilla or flavored

Yogurt, Greek, fat-free (or other plain
  fat-free yogurt)

Meat and Fish

Shop for a good selection of lean meats and seafood. These are my favorites.

Pork tenderloin

Wild salmon fillets

Shrimp

Turkey, lean ground

Turkey breast, skinless slices

Turkey ham or bacon

Fresh Fruits and Vegetables

Keep a wide variety of fruits and vegetables on hand. Below I've listed what I like to keep in my kitchen. The meal plans call for these fruits and vegetables often.

Apples

Bananas

Berries (all types)

Carrots, baby

Cucumbers

Garlic

Grapefruit

Greens, mixed field

Lemons

Lettuce, romaine

Melons

Mushrooms

Onions

Oranges

Peaches

Peppers, red, yellow, or green

Plums

Spinach, baby

Tomatoes

Frozen Foods

Keep your freezer stocked with the following items, replacing them as you use them.

Blueberries, unsweetened

Burgers, turkey (250 calories or less)

Burgers, veggie (150 calories or less; optional)

Chicken breasts, skinless

Dinners, prepared (see page 132 for advice on choosing frozen dinners)

Raspberries, unsweetened

Vegetables, mixed (80 calories or less per cup)

Vegetables, such as broccoli spears, brussels sprouts, cauliflower, green beans, spinach, and sugar snap peas

Waffles, whole grain (80 calories or less per waffle)

Other

Cognac or brandy

Lime juice

Wine, white (such as Chardonnay, Chablis, or Sauterne)

Beverages

Coffee (optional)

Orange juice (calcium-fortified)

Seltzer (optional)

Tea (optional)

Tea, unsweetened iced tea mix (optional)

1,200 CALORIE PLAN Phase 1

DAY 1

BREAKFAST

Whole grain cereal with milk and fruit
³⁄₄ to 1 cup whole grain cereal* topped with:
½ cup fat-free milk
½ medium banana (or ½ grapefruit on the side)

Tea/coffee

*Choose whole grain cereal with 120 calories or less and 3 or more grams of fiber per ³⁄₄ to 1 cup.

AM SNACK

Choose any snack from the 100-Calorie Snack List (page 320).

LUNCH

Tuna Salad over fresh greens
Tuna Salad (page 190) over an unlimited amount of baby spinach leaves or field greens (be sure to choose canned light tuna)

1 mini whole wheat pita*

Water/seltzer/unsweetened iced tea

*Choose mini whole wheat pitas with 70 calories or less per pita.

PM SNACK

Choose any snack from the 100-Calorie Snack List (page 320).

DINNER

Chicken teriyaki over stir-fried vegetables
Chicken: Season a 5-ounce skinless chicken breast with 2 tablespoons low-sodium soy sauce or teriyaki sauce and black pepper to taste. Broil or grill chicken about 12 minutes or until center is no longer pink. Slice into strips.

Vegetables: Coat a pan or wok with cooking spray. Heat 1 teaspoon olive oil in pan over high heat, then toss in vegetables* (½ cup sliced fresh or frozen carrots; 1 cup chopped fresh or frozen broccoli; ½ cup chopped onion; 1 sliced red, yellow, or green pepper). Stir-fry, adding 1 to 2 tablespoons low-sodium teriyaki sauce as you stir, for about 5 minutes or until vegetables are tender. Serve vegetables in a warm bowl with chicken strips on top.

Water/seltzer/unsweetened iced tea

*You may substitute 2 cups frozen mixed vegetables with 80 calories or less per cup.

DAY 2

BREAKFAST

Waffles with vanilla yogurt and berries

1 low-fat frozen waffle (preferably whole grain)* topped with:

6 ounces vanilla (or flavored) fat-free yogurt

2 tablespoons blueberries

1 tablespoon wheat germ

Tea/coffee

*Choose whole grain waffles with 80 calories or less per waffle.

AM SNACK

Choose any snack from the 100-Calorie Snack List (page 320).

LUNCH

Turkey burger with Black Bean Salad

Burger: Cook a 5-ounce lean ground turkey patty* (seasoned to taste) under the broiler, on the grill, or in a nonstick pan. Top the burger with salsa and optional Dijon or yellow mustard. Serve on a bed of an unlimited amount of salad greens.

Black Bean Salad (page 179)

Water/seltzer/unsweetened iced tea

*You may subsitute a frozen turkey burger with less than 250 calories. Or substitute a veggie (garden) burger (150 calories or less) and double the portion of black bean salad.

PM SNACK

Choose any snack from the 100-Calorie Snack List (page 320).

DINNER

Caesar salad with grilled shrimp or chicken

Salad: Place 4 ounces shrimp or sliced skinless chicken breast (grilled, broiled, steamed, or poached) over an unlimited amount of romaine lettuce. Toss with 2 to 4 tablespoons low-calorie Caesar dressing* and sprinkle with 2 tablespoons grated Parmesan cheese.

Water/seltzer/unsweetened iced tea

*Choose Caesar dressing with 80 calories or less per 2 tablespoons.

DAY 3

BREAKFAST

Stuffed western egg-white sandwich

Sandwich: In a nonstick pan coated with cooking spray, sauté ¼ cup chopped green pepper over medium heat until soft. Add 4 whipped egg whites plus 1 chopped slice cooked turkey ham (or bacon). Scramble until cooked through. Stuff into 1 warmed mini whole wheat pita* and top with 2 tablespoons salsa. For a little extra kick, add a few dashes of Tabasco sauce or 1 chopped jalapeño pepper.

Tea/coffee

*Choose mini whole wheat pitas with 70 calories or less per pita.

AM SNACK

Choose any snack from the 100-Calorie Snack List (page 320).

LUNCH

Turkey sandwich with baby carrots

Sandwich: Place 3 ounces cooked skinless turkey breast slices (or lean ham), 1 slice tomato (¼" thick), and an unlimited amount of lettuce between 2 slices reduced-calorie whole grain bread* spread with 1 tablespoon reduced-fat mayonnaise and optional Dijon or yellow mustard.

1 cup baby carrots

Water/seltzer/unsweetened iced tea

*Choose reduced-calorie whole grain bread with 45 calories or less per slice.

PM SNACK

Choose any snack from the 100-Calorie Snack List (page 320).

DINNER

Grilled wild salmon with brussels sprouts

Salmon: Season a 5-ounce wild salmon fillet with 1 teaspoon olive oil and lemon juice, salt, and pepper to taste. Broil, grill, or bake until cooked through. (To save time, you can microwave the salmon on high on a covered plate for 1 to 2 minutes.)

½ cup steamed brussels sprouts or sugar snap peas

1 cup sliced red, yellow, or green pepper

Water/seltzer/unsweetened iced tea

DAY 4

BREAKFAST

Bring-on-the-Morning Smoothie with turkey bacon
    1 serving Bring-on-the-Morning Smoothie (page 180)
    2 slices cooked lean turkey bacon*

Tea/coffee

*You may substitute 1 hard-boiled egg.

AM SNACK

Choose any snack from the 100-Calorie Snack List (page 320).

LUNCH

Open-faced grilled cheese and tomato sandwich with vegetable salad
    Sandwich: Toast 2 slices reduced-calorie whole grain bread.* Top each with tomato slices (¼" thick) and 1 slice reduced-fat American cheese. Place in hot toaster oven for about 1 minute or until cheese melts. Serve warm.

    Salad: Place an unlimited amount of field or mixed greens and fresh vegetables of your choice (broccoli, cauliflower, cucumbers) on a plate. Top with 2 tablespoons canned chickpeas (rinsed and drained). Toss with 1 teaspoon olive oil and 1 tablespoon vinegar or fresh lemon juice.**

Water/seltzer/unsweetened iced tea

*Choose reduced-calorie whole grain bread with 45 calories or less per slice.

**For dressing, you may substitute 2 tablespoons of any low-fat dressing with 40 calories or less per 2 tablespoons.

PM SNACK

Choose any snack from the 100-Calorie Snack List (page 320).

DINNER

Baked Fish with Sweet Carrots
    Baked Fish (page 178)
    Sweet Carrots (page 188)

1 cucumber, sliced

Water/seltzer/unsweetened iced tea

1,200 CALORIE PLAN Phase 1

DAY 5

BREAKFAST

Yogurt with peanut butter toast

6 ounces Greek fat-free yogurt* mixed with:

2 tablespoons raspberries

1 slice toasted whole grain bread** topped with:

1 level teaspoon peanut butter, almond butter, or soy butter

Tea/coffee

*You may substitute 6 ounces of any fat-free flavored yogurt.

**Choose whole grain bread with 80 calories or less per slice.

AM SNACK

Choose any snack from the 100-Calorie Snack List (page 320).

LUNCH

1 serving Wild Salmon with Spicy Salsa* (page 186)

Unlimited fresh spinach leaves or other leafy greens drizzled with optional lemon juice

Water/seltzer/unsweetened iced tea

*You may substitute store-bought salsa with 20 calories or less per 2 tablespoons.

PM SNACK

Choose any snack from the 100-Calorie Snack List (page 320).

DINNER

Vegetable Omelet (page 191)

½ grapefruit

Water/seltzer/unsweetened iced tea

DAY 6

BREAKFAST

Vanilla-cinnamon french toast

French toast: Dip 1 slice whole grain bread* into 2 egg whites whipped with a dash of cinnamon and nutmeg and 1 teaspoon vanilla. Fry in a nonstick pan coated with cooking spray over medium heat until crisp on both sides.

1 tablespoon lite maple syrup

½ grapefruit

Tea/coffee

*Choose whole grain bread with 80 calories or less per slice. Or use 2 slices reduced-calorie bread with 45 calories per slice.

AM SNACK

Choose any snack from the 100-Calorie Snack List (page 320).

LUNCH

Cottage cheese with fresh fruit

1 cup fat-free or 1% reduced-fat cottage cheese mixed with:

1 to 2 tablespoons wheat germ

½ cubed cantaloupe (or ½ cup berries, ½ chopped mango, or 1 sectioned grapefruit)

Water/seltzer/unsweetened iced tea

PM SNACK

Choose any snack from the 100-Calorie Snack List (page 320).

DINNER

1 serving Chicken with White Wine and Mushrooms (page 181)

8 asparagus spears, steamed

Water/seltzer/unsweetened iced tea

DAY 7

BREAKFAST

Old-fashioned oatmeal with strawberries

Oatmeal: Prepare ½ cup oatmeal according to package directions with ½ cup fat-free milk and ½ cup water. (Optional: Flavor the oatmeal with cinnamon, nutmeg, or calorie-free artificial sweetener.) Top with:

5 strawberries, sliced or chopped

Tea/coffee

AM SNACK

Choose any snack from the 100-Calorie Snack List (page 320).

LUNCH

Grilled chicken with chickpea salad

Chicken: Grill a 4-ounce skinless chicken breast over high heat until cooked through, 8 to 10 minutes. Transfer to a plate to cool. Slice into strips.

Salad: Chop ½ tomato, ¼ green pepper, ½ cucumber, and 1 celery stalk. Add ¼ cup canned chickpeas (rinsed and drained) and 1 tablespoon chopped fresh parsley. Place over 2 cups baby spinach or lettuce. Top with the grilled chicken and toss with 2 to 4 tablespoons low-calorie dressing.*

Water/seltzer/unsweetened iced tea

*Choose low-calorie salad dressing with 40 calories or less per 2 tablespoons. Or use 1 teaspoon olive oil and 2 to 4 tablespoons vinegar and/or fresh lemon juice.

PM SNACK

Choose any snack from the 100-Calorie Snack List (page 320).

DINNER

Grilled sirloin with tomatoes and balsamic dressing

Steak: Preheat a large skillet or a grill to medium-high heat. Sprinkle a 4-ounce lean sirloin steak (trimmed of all fat) with salt and pepper to taste. Cook to preferred temperature.

Tomatoes: Cut 1 tomato into thick slices and drizzle with 2 to 4 tablespoons plain balsamic vinegar. Enjoy with optional sliced onions.

Steamed spinach: Place 3 cups raw spinach in a steamer or strainer over boiling water and steam 3 to 4 minutes. Season with salt and pepper to taste. Serve warm.

Water/seltzer/unsweetened iced tea

1,500 CALORIE PLAN Phase 1

DAY 1

BREAKFAST

Whole grain cereal with milk and fruit

$3/4$ to 1 cup whole grain cereal* topped with:

1 cup fat-free milk

$1/2$ medium banana (or $1/2$ grapefruit on the side)

Tea/coffee

*Choose whole grain cereal with 120 calories or less and 3 or more grams of fiber per $3/4$ to 1 cup.

AM SNACK

Choose any snack from the 100-Calorie Snack List (page 320).

LUNCH

Tuna Salad over fresh greens

Tuna Salad (page 190) over an unlimited amount of baby spinach leaves or field greens (be sure to choose canned light tuna)

1 mini whole wheat pita*

1 cup fresh pineapple chunks (or $1/2$ mango, 1 orange, or 1 cup berries)

Water/seltzer/unsweetened iced tea

*Choose mini whole wheat pitas with 70 calories or less per pita.

PM SNACK

Choose any snack from the 150-Calorie Snack List (page 322).

DINNER

Chicken teriyaki over stir-fried vegetables

Chicken: Season a 5-ounce skinless chicken breast with 2 tablespoons low-sodium teriyaki sauce and black pepper. Broil or grill chicken about 12 minutes or until center is no longer pink. Slice into strips.

Vegetables: Coat a pan or wok with cooking spray. Heat 1 teaspoon olive oil in pan over medium heat, then toss in vegetables* (1 cup fresh or frozen sliced carrots; 1 cup fresh or frozen chopped broccoli; $1/2$ cup chopped onion; 1 sliced red, yellow, or green pepper). Stir-fry, adding 1 to 2 tablespoons low-sodium teriyaki sauce as you stir, until vegetables are tender, about 5 minutes. Serve vegetables in a warm bowl with chicken strips on top.

1 cup red or green grapes

Water/seltzer/unsweetened iced tea

*You may substitute 2 cups frozen mixed vegetables with 80 calories or less per cup.

DAY 2

BREAKFAST

Waffles with vanilla yogurt and berries

2 low-fat frozen waffles (preferably whole grain)* topped with:

6 ounces vanilla (or flavored) fat-free yogurt

2 tablespoons blueberries (or raspberries)

1 teaspoon wheat germ

Tea/coffee

*Choose whole grain waffles with 80 calories or less per waffle.

AM SNACK

Choose any snack from the 100-Calorie Snack List (page 320).

LUNCH

Turkey burger with Black Bean Salad

Burger: Cook a 5-ounce lean ground turkey patty* (seasoned to taste) under the broiler, on the grill, or in a nonstick pan. Serve on ½ whole wheat hamburger bun** with 1 tablespoon ketchup or BBQ sauce, optional Dijon or yellow mustard, and unlimited lettuce leaves

Black Bean Salad (page 179)

Water/seltzer/unsweetened iced tea

*You may substitute a frozen turkey burger with less than 250 calories. Or substitute a veggie (garden) burger (150 calories or less) and double the portion of black bean salad.

**Choose whole wheat buns with 120 calories or less per bun.

PM SNACK

Choose any snack from the 150-Calorie Snack List (page 322).

DINNER

Caesar salad with grilled shrimp or chicken

Salad: Place 5 ounces shrimp or sliced chicken breast (grilled, broiled, steamed, or poached) over an unlimited amount of romaine lettuce. Toss with 4 tablespoons low-calorie Caesar dressing* and sprinkle with 2 tablespoons grated Parmesan cheese.

1 orange

Water/seltzer/unsweetened iced tea

*Choose Caesar dressing with 80 calories or less per 2 tablespoons.

1,500 CALORIE PLAN Phase 1

DAY 3

BREAKFAST

Stuffed Western egg-white sandwich

Sandwich: In a nonstick pan coated with cooking spray, sauté ¼ cup chopped green pepper over medium heat until soft. Add 4 whipped egg whites, 1 ounce shredded fat-free cheese (or ¾ ounce reduced-fat cheese), and 1 chopped slice cooked lean turkey ham (or turkey bacon). Scramble until cooked through and cheese is melted. Stuff into 1 warmed mini whole wheat pita* and top with 2 tablespoons salsa. For a little extra kick, add a few dashes of Tabasco sauce or 1 chopped jalapeño pepper.

Tea/coffee

*Choose mini whole wheat pitas with 70 calories or less per pita.

AM SNACK

Choose any snack from the 100-Calorie Snack List (page 320).

LUNCH

Turkey-cheese sandwich with baby carrots

Sandwich: Place 3 ounces skinless turkey breast slices (or lean ham), 1 small slice (¾ ounce) fat-free cheese, 2 medium tomato slices (¼" thick), and an unlimited amount of lettuce between 2 slices reduced-calorie whole grain bread* spread with 1 tablespoon reduced-fat mayonnaise and optional Dijon or yellow mustard.

1 cup baby carrots

1 cup blueberries (or ½ cantaloupe)

Water/seltzer/unsweetened iced tea

*Choose reduced-calorie whole grain bread with 45 calories or less per slice.

PM SNACK

Choose any snack from the 150-Calorie Snack List (page 322).

DINNER

Grilled wild salmon with brussels sprouts

Salmon: Season a 6-ounce wild salmon fillet with 1 teaspoon olive oil and lemon juice, salt, and pepper to taste. Broil, grill, or bake until cooked through.

1 cup steamed brussels sprouts (or sugar snap peas)

1 cup sliced red, yellow, or green peppers

1 cucumber, sliced

Water/seltzer/unsweetened iced tea

DAY 4

BREAKFAST

Fruit 'n Nut Muffin with turkey bacon
1 Fruit 'n Nut Muffin (page 182)
2 slices cooked turkey bacon

Tea/coffee

AM SNACK

Choose any snack from the 100-Calorie Snack List (page 320).

LUNCH

Open-faced grilled cheese and tomato sandwich with vegetable salad

Sandwich: Toast 2 slices reduced-calorie whole grain bread.* Top each with tomato slices ($\frac{1}{4}$" thick) and 1 slice reduced-fat American cheese. Place in a hot toaster oven for about 1 minute or until cheese melts. Serve warm.

Salad: Place an unlimited amount of field or mixed greens and fresh vegetables (broccoli, cauliflower, cucumbers) on a plate. Top with $\frac{1}{4}$ cup canned chickpeas (rinsed and drained). Toss with 1 teaspoon olive oil and 1 tablespoon vinegar or fresh lemon juice.

$\frac{1}{4}$ cantaloupe (or 1 peach, plum, or orange)

Water/seltzer/unsweetened iced tea

*Choose reduced-calorie whole grain bread with 45 calories or less per slice.

PM SNACK

Choose any snack from the 150-Calorie Snack List (page 322).

DINNER

Baked Fish with Sweet Carrots
Baked Fish (page 178)
Sweet Carrots (page 188)

Mixed Green Salad: Cover a plate with an unlimited amount of romaine lettuce; $\frac{1}{2}$ cup halved cherry tomatoes; $\frac{1}{2}$ cup chopped red, green, or yellow pepper; $\frac{1}{2}$ cup chopped cucumber; and 2 tablespoons canned chickpeas or beans (rinsed and drained). Toss with 2 to 4 tablespoons low-calorie salad dressing.*

Water/seltzer/unsweetened iced tea

*Choose low-calorie salad dressing with 40 calories or less per 2 tablespoons. Or use 1 teaspoon olive oil and 2 tablespoons balsamic vinegar and/or fresh lemon juice.

DAY 5

BREAKFAST

Yogurt with peanut butter toast

6 ounces Greek fat-free yogurt* mixed with:

½ cup raspberries

1 slice toasted whole grain bread** topped with:

2 level teaspoons peanut butter, almond butter, or soy nut butter

Tea/coffee

*You may substitute 6 ounces of any fat-free flavored yogurt.

**Choose whole grain bread with 80 calories or less per slice.

AM SNACK

Choose any snack from the 100-Calorie Snack List (page 320).

LUNCH

1 serving Wild Salmon with Spicy Salsa (page 186)

Unlimited raw spinach leaves or other leafy greens drizzled with optional lemon juice

1 orange (or 1 apple, 1 peach, or ¼ cantaloupe)

Water/seltzer/unsweetened iced tea

*You may substitute store-bought salsa with 20 calories or less per 2 tablespoons.

PM SNACK

Choose any snack from the 150-Calorie Snack List (page 322).

DINNER

Vegetable Omelet (page 191)

Water/seltzer/unsweetened iced tea

DAY 6

BREAKFAST

Vanilla-cinnamon french toast

French toast: Dip 2 slices whole grain bread* into 2 egg whites whipped with a dash of cinnamon and nutmeg and 1 teaspoon vanilla. Fry in a nonstick pan coated with cooking spray over medium heat until crisp on both sides.

1 tablespoon lite maple syrup

$\frac{1}{2}$ grapefruit (or 1 cup cubed papaya or $\frac{1}{2}$ cup cubed mango)

Tea/coffee

*Choose whole grain bread with 80 calories or less per slice.

AM SNACK

Choose any snack from the 100-Calorie Snack List (page 320).

LUNCH

Cottage cheese with fresh fruit

1 cup fat-free or 1% reduced-fat cottage cheese mixed with:

2 tablespoons wheat germ

1 tablespoon chopped nuts (walnuts, almonds, or pecans)

$\frac{1}{2}$ cantaloupe (or 1 sliced banana, 1 cup berries, 1 sliced pear, 1 sectioned grapefruit, or $\frac{3}{4}$ chopped mango)

Water/seltzer/unsweetened iced tea

PM SNACK

Choose any snack from the 150-Calorie Snack List (page 322).

DINNER

1 serving Chicken with White Wine and Mushrooms (page 181)

8 asparagus spears, steamed

1 serving Parmesan-Pureed Cauliflower (page 185)

Water/seltzer/unsweetened iced tea

DAY 7

BREAKFAST

Old-fashioned oatmeal with berries

Oatmeal: Prepare ½ cup oatmeal according to package instructions with ½ cup fat-free milk and ½ cup water. (Optional: Flavor the oatmeal with cinnamon, nutmeg, or calorie-free artificial sweetener.) Top with:

> 1 teaspoon chopped walnuts (or 1 tablespoon wheat germ)
>
> ½ cup fruit (chopped apple; sliced strawberries; blueberries, raspberries, or blackberries)

Tea/coffee

AM SNACK

Choose any snack from the 100-Calorie Snack List (page 320).

LUNCH

Grilled chicken with chickpea salad

Chicken: Grill a 5-ounce skinless chicken breast over high heat until cooked through, 8 to 10 minutes. Transfer to a plate to cool. Slice into strips.

Salad: Chop ½ tomato, ¼ green pepper, ½ cucumber, and 1 celery stalk. Add ½ cup canned chickpeas (rinsed and drained) and 1 tablespoon chopped fresh parsley. Place over 2 cups baby spinach or lettuce. Top with the grilled chicken and toss with 4 tablespoons low-calorie dressing* or Tahini Dressing (page 189).

Water/seltzer/unsweetened iced tea

*Choose low-calorie salad dressing with 40 calories or less per 2 tablespoons.

PM SNACK

Choose any snack from the 150-Calorie Snack List (page 322).

DINNER

Grilled sirloin with tomatoes and balsamic dressing

Steak: Preheat a large skillet or a grill to medium-high heat. Sprinkle a 6-ounce lean sirloin steak (trimmed of all fat) with salt and pepper to taste. Cook to preferred doneness.

Tomatoes: Cut 1 tomato into thick slices and drizzle with 2 to 4 tablespoons plain balsamic vinegar. Enjoy with optional sliced onions.

Steamed spinach: Place 3 cups raw spinach in a steamer or strainer over boiling water and steam 3 to 4 minutes. Season with salt and pepper. Serve warm.

Water/seltzer/unsweetened iced tea

1,800 **CALORIE PLAN** Phase 1

DAY 1

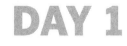

BREAKFAST

Whole grain cereal with nuts and berries

1 cup whole grain cereal* topped with:

½ cup fat-free milk

1 tablespoon chopped nuts (walnuts, almonds, or pecans)

½ cup berries

Tea/coffee

*Choose whole grain cereal with 120 calories or less and 3 or more grams of fiber per 1 cup.

AM SNACK

Choose any snack from the 150-Calorie Snack List (page 322).

LUNCH

Tuna Salad over fresh greens

Tuna Salad (page 190) over an unlimited amount of baby spinach leaves or field greens (be sure to choose canned light tuna)

1 regular-size whole wheat pita*

1 cup fresh pineapple (or ½ mango, 1 orange, or 1 cup berries)

Water/seltzer/unsweetened iced tea

*Choose regular-size whole wheat pitas with 150 calories or less per pita.

PM SNACK

Choose any snack from the 200-Calorie Snack List (page 324).

DINNER

Chicken teriyaki over stir-fried vegetables

Chicken: Season a 5-ounce skinless chicken breast with 2 tablespoons low-sodium soy sauce or teriyaki sauce and salt and pepper to taste. Broil or grill chicken about 12 minutes or until center is no longer pink. Slice into strips.

Vegetables: Spray a pan or wok with cooking spray. Heat 1 teaspoon olive oil in pan over high heat, then toss in vegetables* (1 cup sliced fresh or frozen carrots; 1 cup chopped fresh or frozen broccoli; 1 sliced red, yellow or green pepper; ½ cup chopped onion). Stir-fry, adding 1 to 2 tablespoons low-sodium teriyaki sauce as you stir, until vegetables are tender, about 5 minutes. Serve vegetables in a warm bowl with chicken strips on top.

1 cup boiled soybeans (in the pod, lightly salted)

Water/seltzer/unsweetened iced tea

1,800 **CALORIE PLAN** Phase 1

DAY 2

BREAKFAST

Waffles with vanilla yogurt and berries

2 low-fat frozen waffles (preferably whole grain)* topped with:

6 ounces fat-free vanilla (or flavored) yogurt

2 tablespoons blueberries

½ medium sliced banana

1 teaspoon wheat germ

Tea/coffee

*Choose whole grain waffles with 80 calories or less per waffle.

AM SNACK

Choose any snack from the 150-Calorie Snack List (page 322).

LUNCH

Turkey burger with Black Bean Salad

Burger: Cook a 5-ounce lean ground turkey patty* (seasoned to taste) under the broiler, on the grill, or in a nonstick pan. Serve on 1 whole wheat hamburger bun** with 1 tablespoon ketchup or BBQ sauce, optional Dijon or yellow mustard, and lettuce.

Black Bean Salad (page 179)

Water/seltzer/unsweetened iced tea

*You may substitute a frozen turkey burger with less than 250 calories. Or substitute a veggie (garden) burger (150 calories or less) and double the portion of black bean salad.

**Choose whole wheat buns with 120 calories or less per bun.

PM SNACK

Choose any snack from the 200-Calorie Snack List (page 324).

DINNER

Caesar salad with grilled shrimp or chicken

Salad: Place 6 ounces shrimp or sliced skinless chicken breast (grilled, broiled, steamed, or poached) over an unlimited amount of romaine lettuce. Toss with 4 tablespoons low-calorie Caesar dressing* and sprinkle with 2 tablespoons grated Parmesan cheese and 2 crumbled cooked turkey bacon slices.

1 orange

Water/seltzer/unsweetened iced tea

*Choose Caesar dressing with 80 calories or less per 2 tablespoons.

DAY 3

BREAKFAST

Stuffed Western egg-white sandwich

Sandwich: In a nonstick pan coated with cooking spray, sauté ¼ cup chopped green pepper over medium heat until soft. Add 4 to 5 whipped egg whites, 1 ounce shredded fat-free cheese (or ¾ ounce reduced-fat cheese), and 1 chopped slice cooked turkey ham (or bacon). Scramble until cooked through and cheese is melted. Stuff in 1 warmed mini whole wheat pita (70 calories or less) and top with 2 tablespoons salsa. For a little extra kick, add a few dashes of Tabasco sauce or 1 chopped jalapeño pepper.

½ grapefruit (or 1 orange or tangerine)

Tea/coffee

AM SNACK

Choose any snack from the 150-Calorie Snack List (page 322).

LUNCH

Turkey-cheese sandwich with baby carrots

Sandwich: Place 4 ounces cooked skinless turkey breast or lean ham slices, 1 ounce fat-free cheese (or ¾ ounce reduced-fat cheese), 2 medium tomato slices (¼" thick), and an unlimited amount of lettuce between 2 slices whole grain bread (80 calories or less) spread with 1 tablespoon reduced-fat mayonnaise and optional Dijon or yellow mustard.

1 cup baby carrots

½ cup blueberries (or ½ grapefruit, ½ orange, or ¼ cantaloupe)

Water/seltzer/unsweetened iced tea

PM SNACK

Choose any snack from the 200-Calorie Snack List (page 324).

DINNER

Grilled wild salmon with brussels sprouts and salad

Salmon: Season a 6-ounce wild salmon fillet with 1 teaspoon olive oil and lemon juice, salt, and pepper to taste. Broil, grill, or bake until cooked through.

1 cup steamed brussels sprouts or sugar snap peas

Salad: Cover a plate with an unlimited amount of romaine lettuce. Top with ½ cup halved cherry tomatoes; ½ cup chopped cucumber; ½ cup chopped red, green, or yellow peppers; and ¼ cup canned chickpeas (rinsed and drained). Toss with 2 tablespoons low-calorie salad dressing.

Water/seltzer/unsweetened iced tea

DAY 4

BREAKFAST

Fruit 'n Nut Muffin with Turkey Bacon

> 1 Fruit 'n Nut Muffin (page 182)
> 3 slices cooked turkey bacon*

Tea/coffee

*You may substitute 6 ounces fat-free (flavored) yogurt and 1 tablespoon wheat germ.

AM SNACK

Choose any snack from the 150-Calorie Snack List (page 322).

LUNCH

Open-faced grilled cheese and tomato sandwich with vegetable salad

Sandwich: Toast 2 slices whole grain bread.* Top each with tomato slices (¼" thick) and 1 slice reduced-fat American cheese. Place in hot toaster oven for about 1 minute or until cheese melts. Serve warm.

Salad: Place an unlimited amount of mixed greens and fresh vegetables (broccoli, cauliflower, cucumbers) on a plate. Top with 2 tablespoons canned chickpeas (rinsed and drained) and toss with 1 teaspoon olive oil and 1 tablespoon vinegar or fresh lemon juice.

Frozen banana slices: Slice ½ medium banana and place in freezer for about 1 hour in a zipper-seal bag.

Water/seltzer/unsweetened iced tea

*Choose whole grain bread with 80 calories or less per slice.

PM SNACK

Choose any snack from the 200-Calorie Snack List (page 324).

DINNER

Baked Fish with Sweet Carrots

> Baked Fish (page 178)
> Sweet Carrots (page 188)

1 medium steamed artichoke

2 to 4 tablespoons low-calorie salad dressing* for dipping

1 pear (or 1 apple, ½ cantaloupe, or 1 cup berries)

Water/seltzer/unsweetened iced tea

*Choose low-calorie salad dressing with 40 calories or less per 2 tablespoons.

1,800 **CALORIE PLAN** Phase 1

DAY 5

BREAKFAST

Yogurt with peanut butter toast

    6 ounces Greek fat-free yogurt mixed with:

        1/4 cup raspberries or blackberries

        1 tablespoon wheat germ

    1 slice whole grain toast topped with:

        1 level tablespoon peanut butter, almond butter, or soy butter

Tea/coffee

AM SNACK

Choose any snack from the 150-Calorie Snack List (page 322).

LUNCH

1 serving Wild Salmon with Spicy Salsa (page 186)

Unlimited raw spinach leaves or other leafy greens drizzled with optional lemon juice

1/2 plain baked potato topped with optional 2 tablespoons salsa

Water/seltzer/unsweetened iced tea

*You may substitute any store-bought salsa with 20 calories or less per 2 tablespoons.

PM SNACK

Choose any snack from the 200-Calorie Snack List (page 324).

DINNER

Vegetable Omelet with turkey bacon

    Vegetable Omelet (page 191)

    4 slices cooked lean turkey bacon

1 cup mixed berries (or 1 sliced apple or 1/2 cantaloupe)

Water/seltzer/unsweetened iced tea

DAY 6

BREAKFAST

Vanilla-cinnamon french toast

French toast: Dip 2 slices whole grain bread* into 2 egg whites whipped with a dash of cinnamon and nutmeg and 1 teaspoon vanilla. Fry in a nonstick pan coated with cooking spray over medium heat until crisp on both sides.

2 tablespoons lite maple syrup

1 grapefruit

Tea/coffee

*Choose whole grain bread with 80 calories or less per slice.

AM SNACK

Choose any snack from the 150-Calorie Snack List (page 322).

LUNCH

Cottage cheese with fresh fruit

1 cup fat-free or 1% reduced-fat cottage cheese mixed with:

$1\frac{1}{2}$ cups chopped cantaloupe (or 1 cup mixed berries, 1 chopped mango, or 1 sectioned grapefruit)

2 tablespoons wheat germ

2 tablespoons chopped nuts or seeds (walnuts, almonds, pecans, or sunflower seeds)

Water/seltzer/unsweetened iced tea

PM SNACK

Choose any snack from the 200-Calorie Snack List (page 324).

DINNER

1 serving Chicken with White Wine and Mushrooms (page 181)

8 asparagus spears, steamed

1 serving Parmesan Pureed Cauliflower (page 185)

Mixed green salad: Cover a plate with an unlimited amount of romaine lettuce, $\frac{1}{2}$ cup halved cherry tomatoes; $\frac{1}{2}$ cup chopped cucumber; and $\frac{1}{2}$ cup chopped red, green, or yellow pepper. Toss with 2 tablespoons low-calorie salad dressing.*

Water/seltzer/unsweetened iced tea

*Choose low-calorie salad dressing with 40 calories or less per 2 tablespoons. Or use 1 teaspoon olive oil and 2 to 4 tablespoons vinegar and/or fresh lemon juice.

DAY 7

BREAKFAST

Old-fashioned oatmeal with berries

Oatmeal: Prepare ½ cup oatmeal according to package directions with ½ cup fat-free milk and ½ cup water. Mix in 1 tablespoon chopped walnuts or pecans. (Optional: Flavor the oatmeal with cinnamon, nutmeg, and/or calorie-free artificial sweetener.) Top with:

1 cup berries (or 1 chopped apple)

Tea/coffee

AM SNACK

Choose any snack from the 150-Calorie Snack List (page 322).

LUNCH

Grilled chicken with chickpea salad

Chicken: Grill a 5-ounce skinless chicken breast over high heat until cooked through, 8 to 10 minutes. Transfer to a plate to cool. Slice into strips.

Salad: Chop ½ tomato, ¼ green pepper, ½ cucumber, and 1 celery stalk. Add ¼ cup canned chickpeas (rinsed and drained), ¼ cup canned kidney beans (rinsed and drained), 1 tablespoon sunflower seeds (or 1 tablespoon slivered almonds, chopped walnuts, or toasted pecans), and 1 tablespoon chopped fresh parsley. Place over 2 cups fresh baby spinach or lettuce. Top with the grilled chicken and toss with 4 tablespoons low-calorie salad dressing* or Tahini Dressing (page 189).

Water/seltzer/unsweetened iced tea

*Choose low-calorie salad dressing with 40 calories or less per 2 tablespoons.

PM SNACK

Choose any snack from the 200-Calorie Snack List (page 324).

DINNER

Grilled sirloin with Mozzarella and Tomato Salad

Steak: Preheat a large skillet or a grill to medium-high heat. Sprinkle a 6-ounce lean sirloin steak (trimmed of all fat) with salt and pepper to taste. Cook to preferred doneness.

Mozzarella and Tomato Salad (page 183)

Steamed spinach: Place 3 to 4 cups raw spinach in a steamer or strainer over boiling water and steam 3 to 4 minutes. Season with salt and pepper to taste.

Water/seltzer/unsweetened iced tea

YOUR PHASE 1 EXERCISE ROUTINE AT A GLANCE

In the following pages, you will find small photos of your Phase 1 exercise routine. This routine is no different from that described in detail in Chapter 3. I've included these pages here so you can easily see the routine at a glance. I hope it enables you to start your 3-2-1 fitness journey in the easiest way possible.

WARMUP

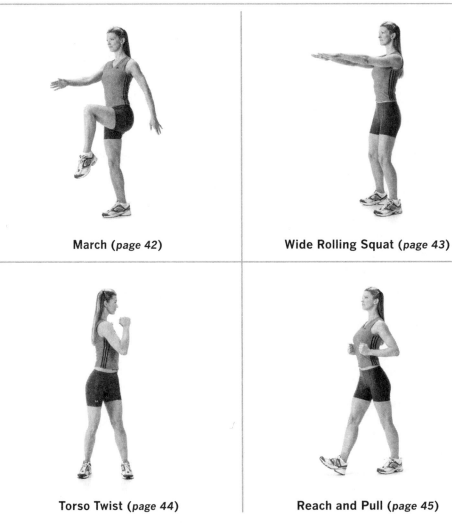

March (*page 42*)

Wide Rolling Squat (*page 43*)

Torso Twist (*page 44*)

Reach and Pull (*page 45*)

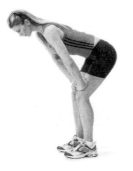

Bend and Round (*page 46*)

ARMS CIRCUIT

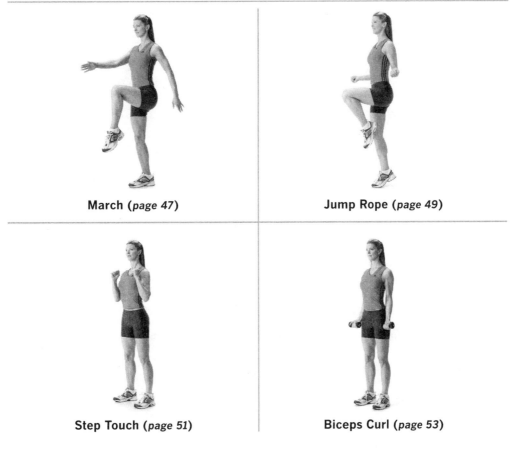

March (*page 47*)

Jump Rope (*page 49*)

Step Touch (*page 51*)

Biceps Curl (*page 53*)

ARMS CIRCUIT *continued*

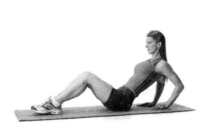

Triceps Dip (*page 55*)

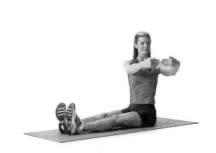

Dandasana Twist (*page 57*)

LEGS AND SHOULDERS CIRCUIT

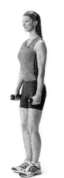

Heel Touch (*page 58*)

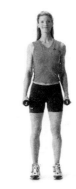

Jacks (*page 59*)

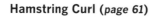

Hamstring Curl (*page 61*)

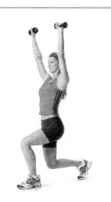

Lunge with Shoulder Press (*page 62*)

LEGS AND SHOULDERS CIRCUIT *continued*

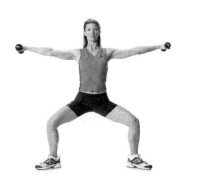

Plié Squat with Shoulder Raise (*page 63*)

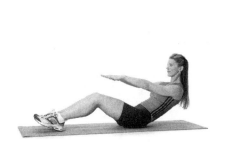

Roll Back (*page 64*)

CHEST CIRCUIT

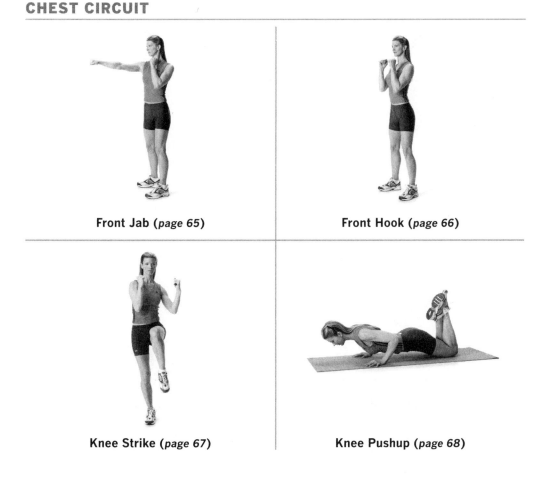

Front Jab (*page 65*)

Front Hook (*page 66*)

Knee Strike (*page 67*)

Knee Pushup (*page 68*)

CHEST CIRCUIT *continued*

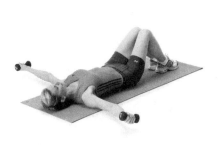

Chest Fly (*page 70*)

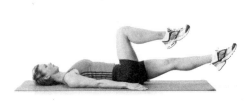

Pilates Bicycle (*page 72*)

BUNS CIRCUIT

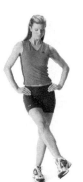

Step Touch with a Soccer Kick (*page 74*)

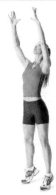

Shoot a Basketball (*page 75*)

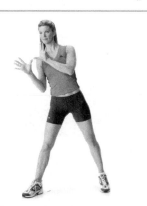

Catch a Football (*page 76*)

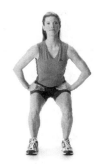

Squat with Leg Lift (*page 77*)

BUNS CIRCUIT *continued*

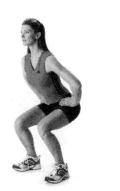

Squat with Knee Lift (*page 79*)

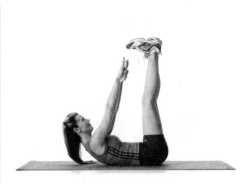

Reverse Curl with Toe Reach (*page 81*)

BACK CIRCUIT

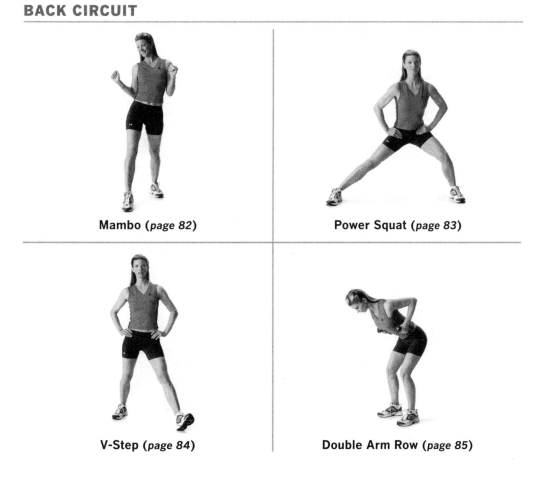

Mambo (*page 82*)

Power Squat (*page 83*)

V-Step (*page 84*)

Double Arm Row (*page 85*)

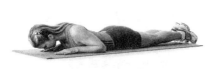

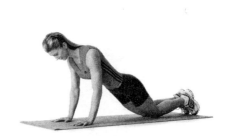

Back Extension (*page 87*)   **Body Plank** (*page 88*)

COOLDOWN

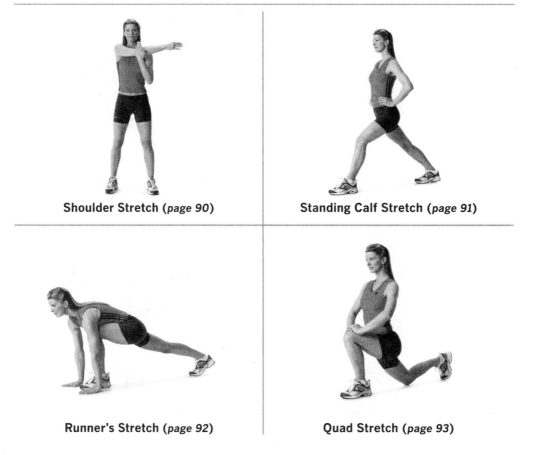

Shoulder Stretch (*page 90*)   **Standing Calf Stretch** (*page 91*)

Runner's Stretch (*page 92*)   **Quad Stretch** (*page 93*)

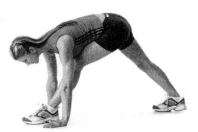

Hamstring Stretch (*page 94***)**

Have you completed your first 3-2-1 Progress Report? Do you have the foods you need in your kitchen? Have you scheduled your exercise sessions into your calendar? If you answered yes to all three, then you're ready to start your 3-2-1 journey today. Enjoy Phase 1. I'll see you at the end of the week!

CHAPTER

9

PHASE 1 RECIPES

14 QUICK AND EASY DISHES THAT YOU'LL LOVE

This weight loss plan is about success, which is why I've tried to keep the number of recipes for Phase 1 to a minimum. The last thing you need when embarking on a weight loss plan is the complication of learning how to cook new meals. It's hard enough to get used to a new way of eating and to learn a new exercise routine, without lots of food preparation on top of it all.

For that reason, most of the meals in the Phase 1 menus require very little in the way of preparation. They are so basic that for many of them, I've included the preparation instructions within the menu plan itself. However, some meals are a bit more involved. In the following pages, you'll find 14 more in-depth recipes that correspond to the Phase 1 meal plans. Most of these recipes are a snap to prepare. In fact, many of them require five or fewer ingredients. I've placed the recipes in alphabetical order to make them easy for you to find and use when you need them. When making them, it's very important that you measure your ingredients and eat the appropriate portion size for your individual calorie plan.

Also, please keep in mind that I have not gone out of my way to restrict salt in these recipes. If you have high blood pressure, and your physician has recommended that you cut back on salt, definitely forgo the salt in these recipes. Instead, try salt substitutes (like Mrs. Dash and Morton Salt Substitute) and experiment with herbs and spices.

BAKED FISH

6 ounces fish (preferably tilapia, black cod, or sole)

1 teaspoon olive oil

Salt and freshly ground black pepper to taste

Fresh or dried Mediterranean herbs (such as rosemary, sage, and oregano) to taste

1. Preheat the oven to 350°F. Brush the fish with the oil and season with the salt, pepper, and herbs. Place in a foil-lined baking dish. Bake for 10 to 12 minutes or until the fish flakes easily.

MAKES 1 SERVING

PER SERVING: 210 calories, 34 g protein, 0 g carbohydrate, 8 g fat (1.5 g saturated), 85 mg cholesterol, 120 mg sodium, 0 g fiber

BLACK BEAN SALAD

Serve this easy salad on a bed of mixed greens.

¼ cup canned black beans, rinsed and drained
¼ cup chopped onion
¼ cup chopped tomato
1 clove garlic, minced
Salt and freshly ground black pepper to taste

1. Combine the beans, onion, tomato, garlic, salt, and pepper in a medium bowl. Stir until well combined.

MAKES 1 SERVING

PER SERVING: 80 calories, 4 g protein, 17 g carbohydrate, 0 g fat, 0 mg cholesterol, 240 mg sodium, 5 g fiber

BRING-ON-THE-MORNING SMOOTHIE

2 cups cleaned fresh or frozen raspberries, blueberries, or strawberries

1 banana

½ cup orange juice

1 tablespoon lime juice

½ cup crushed ice

Mint leaves (optional)

1. In a blender, combine the berries, banana, orange juice, lime juice, and ice and blend until smooth. Pour into 2 glasses and garnish with the mint leaves (if using).

MAKES 2 SERVINGS (1½ CUPS EACH)

PER SERVING: 130 calories, 2 g protein, 31 g carbohydrate, 1 g fat (0 g saturated), 0 mg cholesterol, 0 mg sodium, 5 g fiber

CHICKEN WITH WHITE WINE AND MUSHROOMS

$^3/_4$ teaspoon salt

$^1/_4$ teaspoon ground white pepper

4 boneless, skinless chicken breast halves
($1^1/_4$ to $1^1/_2$ pounds)

$^1/_4$ cup all-purpose flour

2 tablespoons olive oil

8 ounces mushrooms, thinly sliced

$^1/_3$ cup finely chopped shallot or onion

2 tablespoons cognac or brandy

$^1/_2$ cup dry white wine (such as Chardonnay, Chablis,
or Sauterne)

1 cup low-fat chicken broth

1 tablespoon fresh thyme or $^1/_4$ teaspoon dried

1 teaspoon cornstarch mixed with 1 tablespoon water

1. Preheat the oven to 200°F. Mix $^1/_2$ teaspoon of the salt and the pepper in a small dish. Rub the chicken breasts with the mixture. Place the flour in a shallow dish and dredge the breasts in the flour.

2. Heat the oil in a large nonstick skillet over high heat. Add the chicken and reduce the heat to medium-high. Cook, turning once, until browned and the internal temperature reads 160°F on an instant-read thermometer, about 8 minutes. Transfer the chicken to a baking dish, cover loosely with foil, and place in the oven to keep warm. Leave the fat and any crispy particles in the skillet.

3. Add the mushrooms and shallot or onion to the skillet and sauté over medium-high heat until tender, about 5 minutes. Add the cognac or brandy and the wine, increase the heat to high, and sauté for 3 minutes or until the liquid is reduced by half. Add the broth, thyme, and remaining $^1/_4$ teaspoon salt. Bring to a boil and cook for 5 minutes. Whisk in the cornstarch mixture and cook until the sauce forms a glossy syrup, about 1 minute. To serve, place a breast on each of 4 dinner plates and spoon some of the sauce over each.

MAKES 4 SERVINGS

PER SERVING: 330 calories, 43 g protein, 12 g carbohydrate, 9 g fat (1 g saturated), 100 mg cholesterol, 660 mg sodium, 1 g fiber

FRUIT 'N NUT MUFFINS

1¼ cups all-purpose flour

¾ cup quick-cooking oats

½ cup packed brown sugar

¼ cup wheat bran

1 tablespoon baking powder

½ teaspoon ground cinnamon

½ teaspoon ground allspice

¼ teaspoon salt

1 cup halved California seedless grapes

½ cup grated carrots

½ cup fat-free milk

½ cup applesauce

3 tablespoons canola oil

1 egg, beaten

½ cup chopped walnuts

1. Preheat the oven to 350°F. Line a 12-cup muffin pan with paper liners; set aside.

2. Combine the flour, oats, sugar, bran, baking powder, cinnamon, allspice, and salt in a medium bowl and mix well. Add the grapes, carrots, milk, applesauce, oil, egg, and ¼ cup of the walnuts. Stir just until combined.

3. Spoon the batter into the prepared pan (the cups will be very full) and sprinkle with the remaining ¼ cup walnuts. Bake for 20 to 25 minutes or until a toothpick inserted in the center of a muffin comes out clean.

MAKES 12 MUFFINS

PER MUFFIN: 191 calories, 5 g protein, 28 g carbohydrate, 7 g fat (1 g saturated), 18 mg cholesterol, 187 mg sodium, 2 g fiber

MOZZARELLA AND TOMATO SALAD

1 ounce part-skim mozzarella, cut into 2 thin slices

1 tomato, cut into 4 thick slices

2–4 tablespoons balsamic vinegar

Salt and freshly ground black pepper to taste

1 sprig fresh basil

1. Place each slice of mozzarella between 2 slices of tomato and fan out on a plate. Drizzle the vinegar on top. Sprinkle with the salt and pepper and garnish with the basil.

MAKES 1 SERVING

PER SERVING: 140 calories, 8 g protein, 17 g carbohydrate, 5 g fat (3 g saturated), 15 mg cholesterol, 150 mg sodium, 2 g fiber

NO-GUILT GUACAMOLE

1 California avocado

1 medium tomato, quartered

1/4 cup frozen peas, thawed

1/4 cup chopped onion

1 small jalapeño chile pepper, seeded and coarsely chopped (wear plastic gloves when handling)

1–2 tablespoons fresh cilantro leaves

1 tablespoon lime juice

1 teaspoon minced garlic

1/2 teaspoon ground cumin

Salt and freshly ground black pepper to taste

1. Cut the avocado in half lengthwise around the seed. Scoop the flesh into a bowl. Add the tomato, peas, onion, chile pepper, cilantro, lime juice, garlic, and cumin. Season with the salt and pepper.

2. Place the mixture in a food processor or blender and pulse until it reaches the desired consistency.

MAKES 12 SERVINGS (2 TABLESPOONS EACH)

PER SERVING: 55 calories, 1 g protein, 6 g carbohydrate, 3 g fat (0 g saturated), 0 mg cholesterol, 271 mg sodium, 1 g fiber

For a 100-calorie snack: Have 2 tablespoons guacamole with 1 cup mixed raw broccoli and cauliflower florets.

For a 150-calorie snack: Have 3 tablespoons guacamole with 2 cups mixed raw broccoli and cauliflower florets.

For a 200-calorie snack: Have 4 tablespoons guacamole with 2 cups mixed raw broccoli and cauliflower florets and 1 small whole wheat pita, toasted and sliced.

PARMESAN PUREED CAULIFLOWER

3 cups fresh or frozen cauliflower florets

1 clove garlic, minced (optional)

1 teaspoon olive oil (optional)

1 cup frozen mixed vegetables* (optional)

2 tablespoons grated Parmesan cheese

1 teaspoon reduced-fat, soft tub, trans fat–free margarine spread

$\frac{1}{2}$ cup fat-free milk, or to taste

1. If using fresh cauliflower, steam or boil until soft, then drain. If using frozen cauliflower, cook according to package directions and drain. Place in a food processor and puree for 30 seconds or until smooth.

2. If desired, sauté the garlic in the oil over medium heat for about 3 minutes or until soft.

3. Add the sautéed garlic and oil (if using), the vegetables (if using), and the Parmesan and margarine to the cauliflower. Pulse until combined. Slowly add the milk, intermittently pureeing and checking the consistency, adding only enough milk to reach the desired consistency. Serve hot.

MAKES 2 SERVINGS

PER SERVING: 100 calories, 7 g protein, 12 g carbohydrate, 4 g fat (1.5 g saturated), 6 mg cholesterol, 192 mg sodium, 4 g fiber

* Look for frozen vegetables with 80 calories or less per cup.

WILD SALMON WITH SPICY SALSA

You can use store-bought salsa instead of making your own. Serve the salmon and salsa over a generous bed of baby spinach.

1 pint grape or cherry tomatoes, halved

1 cup canned corn, well drained

2 scallions, minced

1 teaspoon olive oil

2 tablespoons balsamic vinegar

Salt to taste

Hot pepper sauce to taste

2 tablespoons onion-flavored mustard

4 wild salmon fillets (4 to 6 ounces each)

1. Preheat the broiler. To make the salsa, in a small bowl, combine the tomatoes, corn, scallions, olive oil, and 1 tablespoon of the vinegar; add the salt and hot pepper sauce.

2. In a small bowl, stir together the mustard and remaining 1 tablespoon vinegar.

3. Place the salmon fillets on a broiler pan skin side up. Broil 4 to 6 inches from the heat for 2 minutes. Turn the fillets and brush with the mustard mixture. Broil until just slightly opaque in the center, 3 to 4 minutes longer depending on thickness. Serve with the salsa.

MAKES 4 SERVINGS

PER SERVING: 330 calories, 34 g protein, 13 g carbohydrate, 15 g fat (2 g saturated), 90 mg cholesterol, 330 mg sodium, 2 g fiber

STRAWBERRY YOGURT FREEZE

2 containers (8 ounces each) fat-free strawberry yogurt
1 pint strawberries, cleaned
1 teaspoon grated orange peel (optional)

1. Mix the yogurt (if it's not premixed) and spoon into an ice cube tray. Freeze until completely solid, 3 to 4 hours.

2. Place the cubes in a food processor and pulse until finely chopped. Add the strawberries and orange peel (if using) and process just until almost smooth. Serve immediately.

MAKES 3 SERVINGS (1 CUP EACH)

PER SERVING: 102 calories, 7 g protein, 38 g carbohydrate, 0 g fat (0 g saturated), 10 mg cholesterol, 101 mg sodium, 2 g fiber

For a 100-calorie snack: Enjoy 1 serving of the yogurt freeze.

For a 150-calorie snack: Enjoy 1 serving of the yogurt freeze with 2 heaping tablespoons of fat-free whipped topping.

For a 200-calorie snack: Have the yogurt freeze with 2 heaping tablespoons of fat-free whipped topping and $\frac{1}{2}$ cup berries on the side. Or enjoy $1\frac{1}{2}$ servings of the yogurt freeze with 2 heaping tablespoons of fat-free whipped topping.

SWEET CARROTS

1 cup sliced peeled carrots

2 teaspoons lemon juice

1 teaspoon olive oil

1 teaspoon sugar

1. Cook the carrots in a saucepan of boiling water until tender, about 10 minutes. Drain and toss with the lemon juice, oil, and sugar.

MAKES 1 SERVING

PER SERVING: 110 calories, 1 g protein, 17 g carbohydrate, 5 g fat (0.5 g saturated), 0 mg cholesterol, 85 mg sodium, 3 g fiber

TAHINI DRESSING

This slightly tangy dressing tastes fantastic with chickpea salad.

2 tablespoons plain fat-free yogurt

2 teaspoons tahini (sesame paste)

1½ teaspoons lemon juice

¼ teaspoon ground cumin

¼ clove garlic, minced

⅛ teaspoon coarse salt

Pinch of ground red pepper

1. Whisk the yogurt, tahini, lemon juice, cumin, garlic, salt, and red pepper in a small bowl until smooth.

MAKES 1 SERVING

PER SERVING: 80 calories, 4 g protein, 6 g carbohydrate, 5 g fat (0.5 g saturated), 0 mg cholesterol, 270 mg sodium, 0 g fiber

TUNA SALAD

Enjoy this salad spread over a split, toasted pita bread or scoop it onto a bed of baby spinach or field greens and enjoy with warm pita bread on the side. Do not use extra salad dressing. Be sure to buy canned light tuna because white albacore has been shown to contain too much mercury.

1 can (6 ounces) water-packed light tuna, drained
$\frac{1}{2}$ cup chopped celery
$\frac{1}{2}$ small green apple, cored and chopped
1 tablespoon reduced-fat mayonnaise
1 small scallion, chopped
Freshly ground black pepper to taste

1. In a small bowl, combine the tuna, celery, apple, mayonnaise, scallion, and pepper.

MAKES 1 SERVING

PER SERVING, WITHOUT PITA OR GREENS: 230 calories, 36 g protein, 13 g carbohydrate, 3 g fat (1 g saturated), 40 mg cholesterol, 650 mg sodium, 2 g fiber

VEGETABLE OMELET

½ cup chopped red, green, or yellow pepper
½ cup chopped or sliced mushrooms
¼ cup sliced onion
1 egg, whipped
5 egg whites or 1½ cups egg substitute
½ cup shredded fat-free cheese
Salt and freshly ground black pepper to taste

1. Coat a nonstick pan with cooking spray and heat over medium heat. Sauté the bell pepper, mushrooms, and onion until soft. Add the egg and egg whites to the pan and cook until browned on one side. Sprinkle with the cheese. Fold over and cook until the cheese melts. Season with the salt and pepper.

MAKES 1 SERVING

PER SERVING: 285 calories, 46 g protein, 11 g carbohydrate, 5.5 g fat (1.5 g saturated), 223 mg cholesterol, 792 mg sodium, 2 g fiber

PART III

Phase 2

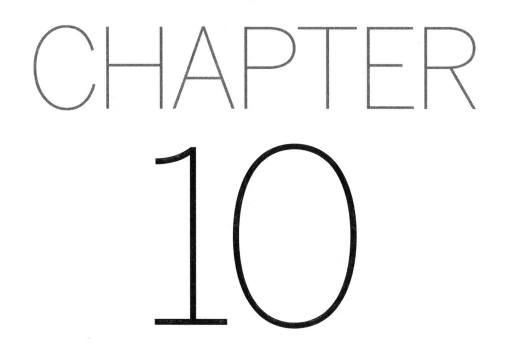

CHAPTER
10

ABOUT PHASE 2

WHAT YOU NEED TO KNOW
BEFORE YOU START

Congratulations on completing the first phase of your 3-2-1 journey. By now you have already seen fantastic results—and you're just one week into this new way of living.

Phase 2 of your journey lasts until you lose all the weight you want. During this phase, you will continue to eat, move, and live by all of the 3-2-1 principles that you incorporated into your life during Phase 1. Phase 2 differs from Phase 1 in three ways.

A ramped-up exercise routine and schedule. Once you feel physically ready, progress to the more challenging Phase 2 exercise routine, shown at a glance on page 258. (If you were out of shape before starting 3-2-1, stick with the Phase 1 routine until you build the fitness required for the Phase 2 routine.) In addition, at some point during Phase 2 (again, only once you are physically ready), you will add a fourth day of exercise to your weekly repertoire. The additional day of exercise coupled with the more rigorous routine will help to challenge your body and burn more calories.

An expanded Treat List. In Phase 1, your Treat List was small and contained 19 indulgent fun foods that were also *healthy*. The dark chocolate, various types of fruit, and wine contained health-improving phytochemicals; the ice cream and pudding supplied you with calcium; and the popcorn had whole grain goodness. I kept the Phase 1 Treat List short and healthy for a number of reasons. First, I wanted Week 1 to be packed with as much nutrition as possible—a powerful springboard for long-term success. Second, I wanted to make you aware that healthy indulgences can be satisfying and delicious so that you're encouraged to choose them indefinitely. Finally, I've found that many weight loss clients—at least in the beginning—find it easier to hold themselves to the right treat portions if they don't have a huge variety of foods to tempt them.

After spending a week with this limited Treat List, however, you're ready to incorporate many more personal favorites. Your Phase 2 Treat List contains all of the nutritious treats from Phase 1 as well as additional treats that still taste decadent but have less nutritional value than the delicious treats you enjoyed last week. Because most of what you eat for 3-2-1 will be incredibly healthy, you can stand to treat yourself to a small amount of not-so-healthy food each day. It won't impede your weight loss at all. As I've said before, treating yourself to a portion-controlled serving of *any* delicious food— whether it be potato chips, ice cream, cookies, or a latte—reduces the feeling of deprivation that causes you to abandon dieting all together and eat these foods 24/7. So indulge without guilt! Nothing is off-limits. Eat your treat at the time of day you most need it. Your treat is optional. If you don't need your treat on a given day, you may skip it. As I mentioned in Phase 1, you can have one portion of fruit or starch or 2 ounces of protein in its place. Or, if you are not hungry, you can skip it altogether.

High-quality starch with dinner. In Phase 1, you did not see rice, pasta, potatoes, bread, or any other starchy carbohydrates in the dinner menus. As I've mentioned, many of the dieters I've counseled tended to overeat these foods at night. Phase 1 is designed to help you to break this bad habit, teaching you to satisfy your nighttime urge to chew with low-calorie, low-starch vegetables such as broccoli and asparagus. Now you are ready to reintroduce high-quality starchy foods to your plate. In most of the dinners in Phase 2 (a few of the 1,200-calorie meal plan options are exceptions to this rule), you will see one of the following high-quality starchy carbs with your meal: brown rice, wild rice, baked white or sweet potatoes, corn, peas, whole wheat couscous, whole grain bread, or whole wheat pasta. I call these choices *high-quality* because that's exactly what they are. Unlike refined starches (white rice, couscous made from refined grain, bread made from refined flour), these whole grains and starchy vegetables contain health-promoting fiber, vitamins, minerals, and phytochemicals.

MAKE THE MOST OF PHASE 2

In Chapter 11, you will find two weeks' worth of menus for the three different calorie levels: 1,200 calories, 1,500 calories, and 1,800 calories. As with Phase 1, each of the calorie plans follows the same format. As with Phase 1, you may either follow these meal plans in the order I've suggested, or you may mix and match breakfasts, lunches, and dinners to suit your tastes and lifestyle. Also:

- Do not have a red meat dish more than twice a week.

- Use the same substitution guidelines (page 128) to modify the meal plan if you are vegetarian or lactose intolerant.

- Feel free to enjoy and integrate any of the meals from Phase 1.

Below, you will find specific advice for modifying the Phase 2 menus to your personal tastes and lifestyle.

Substitute high-quality starch as needed. If you glance over the menus, you'll see that I've included many different types of high-quality starch with your meals. If you are the type of person who loves one type of starch—say you are a pasta person or a potato person—it's okay to substitute your favorite starch for the starch you see listed for that day's dinner. Use this rule of thumb in making your portion substitution. You may swap ½ medium baked white or sweet potato for:

1 ear of corn (or ¾ cup canned or frozen corn) or

¾ cup frozen or canned peas or

½ cup cooked whole wheat pasta, brown rice, wild rice, or whole wheat couscous

Substitute vegetables as needed. Any nonstarchy vegetable listed on the plan may be replaced with the same amount of any of the following vegetables: asparagus, beets, broccoli, brussels sprouts, cabbage, carrots, cauliflower, celery, cucumbers, eggplant, green beans, greens (collard, mustard, and turnip), kale, kohlrabi, leeks, lettuce, mushrooms, okra, onions, pea pods, peppers, spinach, sugar snap peas, Swiss chard, tomatoes, water chestnuts, or zucchini.

Use frozen dinners as needed. Keep your freezer stocked with frozen dinners that meet the calorie requirements of your plan. As with Phase 1, you will choose frozen dinners based on the calorie breakdown of your meal plan. Unlike Phase 1, you can now choose dinners that include high-quality starch (brown rice, whole wheat pasta, etc.) or serve this starch on the side. Most frozen dinners feature refined grains rather than whole grains. If you can find a frozen dinner with whole grains or a high-quality starch (whole grain pasta, brown or wild rice, whole wheat couscous, peas, corn, winter squash, or potato) consider it a bonus. If not, don't sweat it. A refined grain every once in a while is perfectly okay. Use this guide when choosing frozen dinners.

1,200-calorie plan: Choose any entrée with 350 calories or less.

1,500-calorie plan: Choose any entrée with 400 calories or less. Serve with 1 cup baby carrots or half a grapefruit.

1,800-calorie plan: Choose any entrée with 400 calories or less. Serve with 1 cup baby carrots *and* an unlimited amount of fresh or frozen steamed vegetables (such as cauliflower, peppers, sugar snap peas, green beans, or broccoli) topped with 4 tablespoons grated Parmesan cheese.

Don't forget your 3-minute meal. During Phase 2, you may round out the 3-minute meal from Phase 1 with a high-quality starch. Here's how: Place as much as an entire bag of prewashed salad greens on a dinner plate. Drain a 5-ounce can of light tuna (packed in water), chicken breast, or wild salmon and place on the greens. Toss with 2 tablespoons low-calorie dressing of your choice. (*Note:* In Phase 1, I allowed you up to 4 tablespoons of dressing. To make room for the starch, you will cut back on the dressing now.) Enjoy one mini whole wheat pita (no more than 70 calories) on the side.

If you are following the 1,500-calorie plan, add 1 ounce crumbled feta cheese or 1 ounce grated reduced-fat hard cheese.

If you are following the 1,800-calorie plan, add 2 tablespoons chopped nuts or seeds (any type).

YOUR FAMILY FAVORITES ON 3-2-1

If you need more variety to remain motivated, look for recipes in cookbooks, *Prevention* magazine, and online. Pull out your own collection of recipes. You can turn almost any recipe into a 3-2-1 recipe by following these pointers.

Follow the calorie guidelines for your plan, listed again for your convenience below. If you don't know the calorie information for a specific recipe, consult a local hospital or nutrition consultant. Some of them—for a fee—offer nutritional counseling services that will analyze recipes for you. Some online sites (such as www.calorie-count.com/calories/recipe_analysis.php) will do this for you as well.

Calorie Breakdowns by Plan

Below you will find the calorie breakdowns for each plan. Understanding your breakdown can help when certain foods are not available or practical. Use these breakdowns to choose frozen dinners or alter 3-2-1 meals to fit your personal tastes.

1,200-Calorie Plan

Breakfast: 200 calories	**Lunch:** 300 calories	**Dinner:** 350 calories
AM Snack: 100 calories	**PM Snack:** 100 calories	**Treat:** 150 calories

1,500-Calorie Plan

Breakfast: 250 calories	**Lunch:** 400 calories	**Dinner:** 450 calories
AM Snack: 100 calories	**PM Snack:** 150 calories	**Treat:** 150 calories

1,800-Calorie Plan

Breakfast: 300 calories	**Lunch:** 450 calories	**Dinner:** 550 calories
AM Snack: 150 calories	**PM Snack:** 200 calories	**Treat:** 150 calories

Replace refined grains with whole grains and other high-quality starches. Use whole wheat couscous (usually available in health food stores and some grocery stores) instead of regular couscous; 100 percent whole grain bread instead of white; brown or wild rice instead of white; and baked or roasted potatoes instead of fried. See "Specific Advice about Starch" (page 200) for additional advice about whole grain options.

Swap fatty protein sources for lean protein. Whenever possible, substitute egg whites for whole eggs, fat-free milk for whole, reduced-fat or fat-free cheese for regular, and fish or skinless chicken or turkey breast for fattier red meats.

Enjoy low-contaminant fish. As a nutritionist, I love the fact that fish is low in fat and high in protein. Problem is, some types of fish are also loaded with mercury and other contaminants like PCBs, dioxins, and pesticides. Although these contaminants will not affect your weight loss, they do affect your health. For that reason, I strongly advise you to avoid the following high-mercury fish: swordfish, shark, tilefish, and king mackerel (little mackerel is fine). Tuna is also not great, so limit your consumption of tuna steaks. When it comes to canned tuna, you're better off with chunk light than with albacore, or white. Chunk light has significantly less mercury.

You also want to limit your intake of fish highest in PCBs, dioxins, and pesticides, such as bluefish, wild striped bass, American eel, and farm-raised Atlantic salmon.

For more information, visit Oceans Alive (www.oceansalive.org), a great Web site that provides a pocket guide to seafood that you can print out and take with you to the supermarket or restaurant. You'll also find useful information on many more fish varieties.

Reduce overall fat content whenever possible. Experiment with reducing added oil, butter, margarine, salad dressings, and other fats. Often, a recipe will taste just as delicious without them (and you'll finally be able to taste the vegetables on your salad).

SPECIFIC ADVICE ABOUT STARCH

I'm sure you're happy to learn that most Phase 2 dinners include a high-quality starch. Be aware, however, that the portions of starch that I've suggested on these menus are probably smaller than what you may be used to eating. For example, for the 1,200- and 1,500-calorie plans, you eat a half—*not a whole*—baked potato with dinner. Similarly, the ½ to ¾ cup of pasta or rice may be much less than what you used to eat before you switched to 3-2-1 eating.

These are *healthful* portions and will help your weight loss efforts. On this plan, I've made every attempt to satisfy your hunger by including digestion-slowing protein and lots and lots of nonstarchy vegetables. The protein serving for each meal uses up a lot of precious calories. You need these protein calories to get from meal to meal without feeling ravenous. But to make up for these calories, your high-quality starch portions must shrink.

If you are modifying your family favorites for 3-2-1 success, you will need some pointers for picking whole grain foods. Compared to refined grains (white flour, for example), whole grains house more nutrients, antioxidants, and fiber. Your body typically absorbs them more slowly than refined grains, an effect that steadies blood sugar levels and insulin. This helps you to feel satisfied on fewer calories.

To choose whole grains, look for products made from:

Amaranth	Flour, whole wheat
Barley, whole grain	Millet
Corn on the cob, corn kernels, or pop-corn (*Note:* Cornmeal is *not* a whole grain)	Oats
	Quinoa
Couscous, whole wheat	Rice, brown or wild
	Wheat berries

Choosing whole grains can be tricky, as food marketers have become quite skilled at making refined foods sound healthy. Don't be fooled, for example, by products that claim to be made from *wheat* or to be *multigrain* or *7-grain*. The word *multigrain* only means that different types of grains were used; they may be whole grains or refined grains. And know that phrases like *stoned wheat*, *cracked wheat*, and *wheat flour* do not guarantee the presence of whole grain.

Always check the product's ingredients list to ensure that one of the first few ingredients contains the word *whole* in front of the grain mentioned. Oats are an exception, as they are automatically whole grain, even after processing.

Also, look for a whole grain stamp that often appears on a food's packaging. The Whole Grain Council allows manufacturers to place a stamp on their packaging that says *Whole Grain* if the product contains a half serving (8 grams) or more of whole grains per serving. They can use a stamp that says *100% Whole Grain* if all the grains used are whole and provide a full serving of whole grains per serving.

PHASE 2 RESTAURANT OPTIONS

Your Phase 2 meal options are even more convenient and flexible than Phase 1's because I've incorporated more options for eating out and ordering in. For example, on Day 6, you'll make a black bean burrito for dinner that requires no more preparation than removing it from its package and putting it into your microwave or toaster oven. On Day 9, you can order Chinese food for lunch using the ordering suggestions listed in the meal.

Most other meal items require a small amount of prep work on your part. But, as with Phase 1, you can modify just about all of them for restaurant ordering. To follow the Phase 2 meals at your favorite restaurant, simply order a restaurant meal similar to a meal you find on the plan. You probably won't be able to order exactly what is prescribed here, but you can get close. Use these tips.

- Ask for sauce on the side and use as little of it as possible.

- Ask for low-calorie salad dressing on the side. Use only 2 tablespoons or less. If low-calorie dressing is not available, ask for olive oil and vinegar, using 1 teaspoon oil with unlimited vinegar (or fresh lemon juice).

- Eyeball the size of the meal that comes to your table—if need be, reduce it accordingly. Use the following as a basic rule of thumb for judging the size of restaurant portions.

  Meat: 1 ounce is the size of a matchbox. 3 ounces is the size of a deck of cards.

  Fish: 3 ounces is the size of a checkbook.

  Cheese: 1 ounce is the size of four dice.

  Pasta, rice, or other grain: ½ cup is the size of half a tennis ball.

• If you are eating at a family-style restaurant or fast-food restaurant, ask for the nutritional information for the dishes you are interested in ordering. Most franchise restaurants keep this information handy and will supply it upon request. Use it to figure out the number of calories for any given dish. This will give you a good idea of how much food to immediately put in a takeout container when your dinner is served.

In the following pages, you'll find good 3-2-1 restaurant options taken from the Phase 2 meal plan and modified for restaurant eating.

Breakfast

Broccoli and mushroom omelet with toast: Order an egg-white or egg-substitute omelet. Ask for any vegetables the restaurant offers. Have one slice of whole grain toast and eat it dry. Have any amount of coffee or tea. The restaurant probably won't have the turkey bacon suggested on the 1,500- and 1,800-calorie plans, so be prepared to skip it.

    Whole grain cereal with berries: Order any small box of whole grain cereal. Ask for ½ cup berries (or whatever fruit the restaurant offers) and ½ cup fat-free milk. If you are on the 1,500- or 1,800-calorie plan, either take nuts with you (the restaurant probably won't have them) or be prepared to go without.

    Hard-boiled egg with toasted English muffin and peanut butter: Most restaurants will serve this almost exactly as it's described in your meal plan. Settle for a refined English muffin if the restaurant doesn't offer whole wheat. Make sure to eat only half of it if you are following the 1,200-calorie plan. If you are on the 1,500- or 1,800-calorie plan, eat 1 cup of whatever sliced fruit the restaurant offers or one whole fruit (banana, orange, or apple).

    Cantaloupe with cottage cheese and slivered almonds: This is another meal that you should be able to easily order at any restaurant. Ask for ¼ of a cantaloupe, ½ cup reduced-fat cottage cheese (a large dollop), and 1 tablespoon slivered almonds (take your own if you know your restaurant doesn't have them). If you're on the 1,500- or 1,800-calorie plan, you may also want to pack your own raisins, sunflower seeds, and/or wheat germ.

    Sunnyside-up egg on whole grain toast: Order this straight from your 3-2-1 meal plan. If the restaurant doesn't offer reduced-fat spread, eat the toast dry. If you are following the 1,800-calorie plan, order 1 cup of any type of sliced fruit the restaurant offers.

Lunch

Vegetable bean soup with salad: Order a bowl of any noncreamy vegetable soup along with a mixed salad (omit cheese, croutons, and other high-fat or high-calorie salad ingredients). Dress the salad with plain balsamic vinegar.

Steamed Chinese food: Order this eat-out meal as described in your meal plan.

Caesar salad with grilled shrimp or chicken: Omit any croutons that come with the salad and request dressing on the side. Dress it with 1 tablespoon dressing of your choice or (bonus points) plain balsamic vinegar.

Dinner

Grilled fish with wild rice and snow peas: Order the same amount of grilled fish detailed in your meal plan, choosing whatever type of fish the restaurant offers. Request

---

ASK**JOY**

Can I Eat All the Raw Vegetables I Want?

You may have tried diets that provided you with an "unlimited food list." You were allowed to eat these foods—usually raw vegetables—in whatever quantities you wanted. Can you do the same on the 3-2-1 plan?

I'm somewhat hesitant to say yes, and here's why: I'd like you to learn to stop munching throughout the entire day and instead learn to eat when it's appropriate. With the 3-2-1 program, you eat every 4 to 5 hours. Thus, another meal or snack is right around the corner—you'll never go hungry.

That said, I know that unlimited food lists work really well for some people. Try to follow 3-2-1 for a week and see if you can do without an unlimited snack list. If you do well, you probably don't need the unlimited food option. If you continue to struggle, then by all means incorporate a few unlimited foods. Here's how: When you feel like you just can't get from one meal to the next without putting something in your mouth, do the following.

Turn to no-calorie options first. Try to calm the craving with sugarless gum (up to a pack a day) or by drinking regular or decaf coffee, black tea, green tea, or herbal tea.

Use low-calorie options second. If the gum and/or tea does not satisfy your urge to eat, then go ahead and have some plain (no dip or dressing) raw, nonstarchy vegetables such as sliced bell peppers, celery, broccoli, or cauliflower.

---

steamed plain vegetables with your fish entrée and add a side salad dressed with plain balsamic vinegar and ½ cup steamed rice (or ½ plain baked potato). If the restaurant offers brown or wild rice, great! If not, settle for white.

Grilled turkey burger with mixed green salad: Order exactly as your meal plan describes, but skip the fries since the restaurant's version will probably be fried. Use low-calorie dressing on the salad, if possible, or a dash of olive oil and an unlimited amount of vinegar.

Barbecued grilled chicken with spinach and corn on the cob: You should be able to get this dish almost exactly as your meal plan prescribes (be sure to request no butter on the corn). If corn on the cob is not in season, substitute ½ cup of another starch. You'll probably be served more chicken than your meal plan calls for, so if you're not ravenous, be prepared to put some into a takeout container.

Chicken any which way: You probably won't find a number of specific 3-2-1 chicken recipes at a restaurant, but consider any grilled or baked chicken breast fair game (as long as it is skinless). Order it with a mixed green salad (dressed with a dash of olive oil and unlimited vinegar) and a side of plain steamed vegetables. If you are on the 1,500- or 1,800-calorie plan, you can also have ½ cup rice, ½ baked potato, or another starch.

Broiled pork tenderloin with baked potato and vegetables: Use your meal plan to ensure that you eat the right portions (remember: you get only half a potato on the 1,200-calorie plan), but you should be able to find this menu verbatim at many restaurants. Your tenderloin will probably come in a size much larger than your menu calls for, so be prepared to eat only half of it.

HOW TO SURVIVE VACATIONS, HOLIDAYS, AND OTHER CHALLENGES

If you have a lot of weight to lose, you may very well need to remain in Phase 2 for several months. That means you will follow Phase 2 while on vacation, through the holidays, and through a number of other situations that will challenge your resolve to stick with the program.

To successfully follow 3-2-1 during tough times, use this advice.

Try to lose, but be happy to plateau. No matter the challenge, try to stick as closely to the plan as possible. Try to follow 3-2-1 eating and exercising in the same way you do at any other time of year—and try to lose the same amount of weight you usually lose each week. At the same time, be *happy* about managing to maintain your results. In reality, you simply may not be able to continue to lose weight during the holidays or while you travel. Don't beat yourself up over this. As soon as the challenging time ends, recommit yourself to 3-2-1 and look forward to your continuing success.

Build in a few planned "cheats." When on vacation, try to stick with 3-2-1 eating most of the time. For your enjoyment (you *are* on vacation, after all!), allow yourself a couple of indiscretions. Perhaps you might allow yourself to enjoy:

- A single portion of dessert following two healthy, portion-controlled dinners during a week of vacation.

- One (or two—if you must) meals "off." In other words, when you order, you may eat one reasonable portion of whatever you want. Try not to include dessert with this option.

Try to make up for these splurges by omitting your treat on the other days of your vacation (plus, try to do some extra exercise). Planning for these splurges keeps you in control. You'll be less likely feel guilty, which helps to prevent you from abandoning the plan altogether.

Move up a meal plan for a short period of time. If you are following the 1,200- or 1,500-calorie plan, consider moving up one level to provide yourself with more food to chew on for a short time. Know that this move may cause a temporary plateau or slower weight loss. In making this choice ahead of time, however, you stay in control, so you can feel good about your choices rather than guilty.

3·2·1
SUCCESS STORY
Peggy Shackleton

Age: 41
Accomplishment: Lost 15 pounds in four weeks

Q: How did you gain the excess weight?

A: I am a busy mother of two boys, ages 2 and 11, and I work a desk job. I've always struggled with weight loss. I was in good shape in college when I had no car and had to walk a couple of miles a day, but I have steadily gained weight since then. I lost 20 pounds right before getting pregnant at age 39—the surprise of my life, but I wouldn't change it for the world! Losing 20 right before pregnancy was perfect because that was about what I gained. I got the weight off right after my pregnancy, but then it came back on.

Q: What changes have you noticed in your health?

A: I feel great! I've learned so much—this is the best weight loss plan I've ever tried! I have noticed a dramatic difference in my health, energy, and physical fitness. I can feel the difference in my flexibility, strength, and endurance. It's staggering to me. The first three weeks of exercise were difficult, but now I actually look forward to the days I do it, and I am seeing more results all the time. It keeps me going!

Q: What changes have you noticed in your psychological health?

A: I have noticed a complete overhaul in my mood and overall attitude. I get it—finally, I get it! I feel good when I eat well. I finally realize that I need to exercise to keep up with my busy life. Plus, it feels really good to be taking some time to take care of *me*. It's so great to start the day doing something positive for myself.

Q: How does this weight loss plan compare to others you've tried?
A: This program is perfect for me. I tried Atkins and Weight Watchers in the past and had minimal success. I think this plan has worked because I now see the nutritional mistakes I was making. It's no wonder I wasn't losing! I read every label now. I think the most shocking label (one that I never looked at before) was the Wendy's ranch salad dressing—holy cow!—230 calories, and sometimes I'd get extra! I might as well have been eating a cheeseburger. Plus, I have learned so many things on this program. For example, veggies with low-sodium soy sauce or lemon pepper taste so much better than they do with butter. I don't think I'll ever butter another piece of broccoli again. Also, I learned I can have a whole plate full of veggies for the same calories as a handful of chips, or an entire cup of grapes instead of one slice of bread.

Q: What do you think of the exercises?
A: I love the 3-2-1 workout. I have gotten more success with this workout than with any other I've ever tried. I can see the inches lost in my hips, and my range of motion is expanding every time I exercise.

Q: Overall, what has been your experience with 3-2-1?
A: I love the 3-2-1 concept. It's wonderful and just the right blend of cardio, strength, and abdominal exercise for success. People are already starting to notice my results, and it feels fabulous. I am going to continue with the program until I reach my ultimate goal of 50 pounds. Thank you!

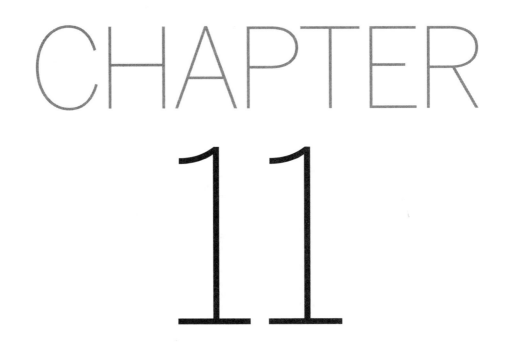

CHAPTER
11

PHASE 2

WHAT TO DO EACH DAY

In the following pages, you will find 14 days' worth of meal suggestions along with small photos that show your Phase 2 exercise routine at a glance. You have everything you need here to continue to lose up to 2 pounds a week until you reach your goal.

As with Phase 1, keep the following in mind when using the meal plans.

- Do not add condiments and other flavorings in amounts above what the plan recommends. Also, if the meal plan calls for reduced-fat mayo, don't use regular mayo instead. If it calls for a packet of sugar, you may *omit* the sugar or use a sugar substitute, but don't add *two* packs of sugar.

- You may drink unlimited amounts of water, seltzer, plain coffee, tea, and other calorie-free beverages. But do not add calories to these drinks by putting cream in your coffee or honey in your tea, for example.

- You may use unlimited amounts of the following seasonings: basil, bay leaves, celery seed, chili powder, chives, cinnamon, cumin, curry, dill, flavoring extracts (such as almond and vanilla), garlic powder, hot pepper sauce, lemon, lemon juice, lemon pepper, lime juice, minced onion, onion powder, oregano, paprika, parsley, pepper, pimiento, low-sodium soy sauce, tarragon, thyme, turmeric, and vinegar.

- Continue to take your multivitamin (and calcium supplements) daily if you've decided supplements are right for you.

- Choose a treat from the Phase 2 Treat Lists as often as daily, eating it at any time of day you most need it.

• For salad dressing, choose a low-calorie brand with 40 calories or less per 2 tablespoons. Or use 1 teaspoon olive oil and 2 to 4 tablespoons vinegar and/or fresh lemon juice.

YOUR 3-2-1 PROGRESS REPORT

Before you embarked on your 3-2-1 journey, you filled out a 3-2-1 Progress Report. I'd like you to take the time to fill out this report again before you start Phase 2 of the program. Rate the following on a scale of 0 to 10 (with 0 indicating the worst you've ever felt and 10 indicating the most fantastic you ever could feel):

How you feel about your health .... ☐

How you feel about your level of energy .... ☐

How you feel about your weight and body .... ☐

How you feel about your level of commitment to losing weight .... ☐

Complete this report again every week for the next three weeks. After that, you should fill it out once a month until you reach your goal. Write down your ratings in a notebook so you can compare notes from rating to rating to see if you are moving in the right direction. As I mentioned before, expect your level of commitment to wax and wane, but if any given rating of your commitment falls below a 5, reread Chapter 4 to help find ways to motivate yourself to move forward. Also focus on the improvements in your other ratings. You will notice, if you compare ratings, that you will most definitely feel better about your weight, energy, and health as your journey continues.

YOUR PHASE 2 GROCERY LIST

The following grocery list will ensure that you have all the food you need on hand. Shop for and stock up on the nonperishables now (you may already have many of them on hand, left over from Phase 1). This list includes suggestions for foods you should consider stocking in your freezer today in case you have unexpected conflicts tomorrow and don't have time to prepare the 3-2-1 lunch or dinner that you planned. If you take the time to stock up on these ingredients now, you'll need to shop for only the fresh items (skinless chicken breast, wild salmon, and fresh vegetables and fruit) as you need them.

Condiments, Spices, and Oils

Keep the following items on hand, replacing them as you use them up.

Barbecue sauce (50 calories or less per 2 tablespoons)

Cheese, Parmesan

Cheese, Romano

Chili powder

Cinnamon, ground

Cooking spray

Cumin, ground

Dressing, ranch, low-calorie

Dressing, salad, low-calorie (40 calories or less per 2 tablespoons, or use olive oil and balsamic vinegar and/or fresh lemon juice)

Garlic powder

Honey

Ketchup

Margarine spread, reduced-fat, soft tub, trans fat–free

Mayonnaise, reduced-fat

Mustard, Chinese (optional)

Mustard, Dijon or yellow

Nutmeg

Oil, canola

Oil, olive

Oil, wheat germ (or use canola oil)

Oregano, dried

Paprika

Parsley, Italian, fresh or dried

Peanut butter

Pepper, black

Pepper, red (cayenne)

Red pepper flakes

Salsa

Salt (or salt substitute)

Soy sauce, low-sodium

Tabasco sauce (optional)

Thyme, dried

Vinegar, balsamic

1,500- and 1,800-Calorie Plans Only

The following spices and sauces are used in your Phase 2 meal plans.

Chutney, plain (or mango salsa)

Cocktail sauce

Dressing, Russian, low-calorie

Dry/Canned Goods

Stock up on the following items, checking levels periodically.

Almonds, slivered

Baking powder

Beans, kidney, canned

Bread, whole grain, reduced-calorie (45 calories or less per slice)

Bread crumbs

Buns, hamburger, whole grain, (150 calories or less per roll)

Buns, hot dog, whole wheat (110 calories or less per bun)

Cereal, cornflakes

Cereal, whole grain (120 calories or less and 3 or more grams of fiber per ¾ to 1 cup)

Chickpeas, canned

Chili, canned or jarred (200 calories or less per cup)

Couscous, whole wheat (110 calories or less per ½ cup cooked)

Flour, all-purpose

Flour, pastry, whole grain

Muffins, English, whole grain

Oatmeal, instant

Pasta, whole wheat (including penne)

Peppers, roasted red, jarred

Pitas, mini, whole wheat (70 calories or less per pita)

Pumpkin, 100% pure, canned

Rice, brown or wild (110 calories or less per ½ cup cooked)

Sauce, tomato or marinara (60 calories or less per ½ cup)

Sauerkraut

Soup, vegetable, canned (125 calories or less per 1 cup)

Soybeans (in the pod)

Sugar

Tomatoes, crushed, canned

Tortillas, whole wheat (100 calories or less) or spinach or sun-dried tomato tortillas

Tuna, light, canned, packed in water

Wheat germ

1,500- and 1,800-Calorie Plans Only

The following staples appear in your Phase 2 meal plans.

Bread, whole wheat (80 calories or less per slice)

Cereal, granola, low-fat

Pita, whole wheat (150 calories or less per pita)

Raisins

Seeds, sunflower

Dairy and Eggs

Try to keep the following on hand.

Cheese, Brie

Cheese, goat

Cheese, mozzarella, reduced-fat

Cheese, Swiss, reduced-fat (40 calories
or less per slice)

Cottage cheese, fat-free or
1% reduced-fat

Cream cheese, soft, reduced-fat

Egg substitute (30 calories or less per
¼ cup) or egg whites

Eggs

Milk, fat-free or 1% reduced-fat milk or
low-fat soy milk

Pudding, fat-free

Sour cream, fat-free or reduced-fat

Yogurt, fat-free, flavored and plain

Meat and Fish

Chicken, ground, lean

Chicken breasts

Chicken tenders or frozen vegetarian
soy nuggets (240 calories or less per
serving)

Hot dogs, turkey, reduced-fat (90
calories or less per dog)

Lox (smoked salmon)

Pork tenderloin

Roast beef, lean, deli-sliced

Scallops, bay

Sirloin steak, chicken, or tofu

Tilapia, wild salmon, or black cod

Turkey bacon, lean

Turkey breast, lean

Turkey, ground, extra-lean

1,500- and 1,800-Calorie Plans Only

The following items come up in your Phase 2 meals.

Fish of your choice

Shrimp, large

Fresh Fruits and Vegetables

The following fruits and vegetables are used in the Phase 2 menus.

Arugula or lettuce

Berries (strawberries and
  blueberries)

Broccoli

Cantaloupe

Cauliflower

Celery

Corn on the cob

Cucumbers

Eggplant

Garlic

Green beans

Greens, mixed field

Lemons

Lettuce, romaine

Mushrooms

Onions (including red onions)

Oranges

Parsley, fresh

Peppers, red, yellow, and green

Potatoes, white

Rosemary, fresh

Scallions

Snow peas

Spinach (including baby)

Tangerines

Tomatoes (including cherry)

Zucchini

1,500- and 1,800-Calorie Plans Only

The following produce items are included in your Phase 2 meals.

Bananas

Carrots, baby

Grapefruit

Grapes, red or green

Potatoes, sweet

Potatoes, white

Frozen Foods

Keep the following frozen items on hand for when you need them.

Berries, unsweetened (or use fresh)

Burritos, black bean and cheese
(280 calories or less per burrito)

Dinners, prepared (see page 197 for
advice on choosing frozen dinners)

Orange juice concentrate

Sausage, soy (40 calories or less per link)

Mixed vegetables (80 calories or less per
1 cup), or use fresh vegetables

Other

Hummus

Tahini

Beverages

Coffee (optional)

Orange juice (calcium-fortified)

Seltzer (optional)

Tea (optional)

Tea, unsweetened iced tea mix
(optional)

Water

1,200 CALORIE PLAN Phase 2

DAY 1

BREAKFAST

Melon with yogurt and wheat germ
½ cantaloupe
6 ounces fat-free flavored yogurt (or ½ cup fat-free or 1% reduced-fat cottage cheese) mixed with:

1 teaspoon wheat germ

Tea/coffee

AM SNACK

Choose any snack from the 100-Calorie Snack List (page 320).

LUNCH

Open-faced turkey Reuben sandwich
Sandwich: Toast 2 slices reduced-calorie whole grain bread*. Top each slice with 2 ounces lean turkey breast (4 ounces total), 1 heaping tablespoon sauerkraut (2 tablespoons total), optional onion slice, and 1 slice reduced-fat Swiss cheese (about 1 ounce total). Bake in 350°F toaster oven until the cheese melts.

Water/seltzer/unsweetened iced tea

*Choose reduced-calorie whole grain bread with 45 calories or less per slice.

PM SNACK

Choose any snack from the 100-Calorie Snack List (page 320).

DINNER

Fish Kebabs with rice
Fish Kebabs (page 274)
½ cup steamed brown or wild rice*

Water/seltzer/unsweetened iced tea

* Choose brown or wild rice with 110 calories or less per ½ cup cooked serving.

DAY 2

BREAKFAST

Toast with cream cheese, tomato, onion. and lox

    2 slices toasted, reduced-calorie, whole grain bread* topped with:
        2 level tablespoons reduced-fat soft cream cheese
        2 slices tomato
        Optional sliced onion
        1 ounce lox (smoked salmon)

Tea/coffee

* Choose reduced-calorie whole grain bread with 45 calories or less per slice.

AM SNACK

Choose any snack from the 100-Calorie Snack List (page 320).

LUNCH

Crispy Chicken Tenders with Honey-Dijon Sauce* (page 271)

1 cup sliced red, yellow, or green pepper

Unlimited celery sticks

Water/seltzer/unsweetened iced tea

* You may substitute frozen vegetarian soy nuggets with 240 calories or less per serving.

PM SNACK

Choose any snack from the 100-Calorie Snack List (page 320).

DINNER

Eggplant Parmigiana with Edamame

    1 serving Eggplant Parmigiana (page 272)
    ³⁄₄ cup boiled soybeans in the pod, lightly salted

Water/seltzer/unsweetened iced tea

1,200 CALORIE PLAN Phase 2

DAY 3

BREAKFAST

Broccoli and mushroom omelet with toast

Omelet: Coat a nonstick pan with cooking spray and heat over medium-high heat. Add ½ cup chopped broccoli and ½ cup sliced (or diced) mushrooms. Sauté until soft. Add 1 cup egg substitute*, brown on both sides, and fold over. Add salt and pepper to taste.

1 slice whole grain toast**, dry

Tea/coffee

* Choose egg substitute with 30 calories or less per ¼ cup. Or substitute 1 egg whipped with 2 egg whites.

** Choose whole grain bread with 80 calories or less per slice. Or substitute reduced-calorie whole wheat bread with 45 calories or less per slice.

AM SNACK

Choose any snack from the 100-Calorie Snack List (page 320).

LUNCH

Vegetable bean soup with salad

2 cups healthy vegetable bean soup*

Salad: Cover a plate with an unlimited amount of romaine lettuce, ½ cup cherry tomatoes, ½ cup chopped red, green, or yellow pepper, and ½ cup chopped cucumber. Toss with 1 tablespoon low-calorie salad dressing.

Water/seltzer/unsweetened iced tea

* Choose canned soup with 125 calories or less per 1 cup.

PM SNACK

Choose any snack from the 100-Calorie Snack List (page 320).

DINNER

Barbecued chicken with spinach and corn on the cob

Chicken: Grill a 5-ounce chicken breast over medium-high heat until cooked through. Top with 2 tablespoons barbecue sauce*.

1 cup steamed spinach

1 medium ear of corn, boiled or grilled, with salt and pepper

Water/seltzer/unsweetened iced tea

* Choose sauce with 50 calories or less per 2 tablespoons.

DAY 4

BREAKFAST

Whole grain cereal with berries
¾ to 1 cup whole grain cereal* topped with:
½ cup fat-free milk
½ cup berries

Tea/coffee

* Choose whole grain cereal with 120 calories or less and 3 or more grams of fiber per ¾ to 1 cup.

AM SNACK

Choose any snack from the 100-Calorie Snack List (page 320).

LUNCH

Turkey hot dog with mixed green salad
1 reduced-fat turkey hot dog* with:
2 tablespoons sauerkraut and unlimited mustard
1 whole wheat hot dog bun**
Salad: Cover a plate with an unlimited amount of romaine lettuce, ½ cup halved cherry tomatoes, ½ cup chopped red, green, or yellow pepper, and ½ cup chopped cucumber. Toss with 2 tablespoons low-calorie salad dressing.

Water/seltzer/unsweetened iced tea

* Choose turkey hot dogs with 90 calories or less per dog.

** Choose whole wheat buns with 110 calories or less per bun.

PM SNACK

Choose any snack from the 100-Calorie Snack List (page 320).

DINNER

Whole wheat pasta primavera with grilled chicken
Pasta: Cook 2 ounces whole wheat linguine or spaghetti according to package directions (makes 1 cup cooked); drain. Steam 1 cup chopped broccoli (fresh or frozen) and ½ cup sliced mushrooms and add to pasta. Stir in ½ cup tomato or marinara sauce* and top with 1 tablespoon grated Parmesan cheese.
2 ounces grilled chicken breast

Water/seltzer/unsweetened iced tea

* Choose sauce with 60 calories or less per ½ cup.

DAY 5

BREAKFAST

Berry-Banana Smoothie with scrambled egg whites

> 1 serving Berry-Banana Smoothie (page 269)
>
> 3 scrambled egg whites with salt and pepper to taste

Tea/coffee

AM SNACK

Choose any snack from the 100-Calorie Snack List (page 320).

LUNCH

Garden tuna wrap

> **Wrap:** Combine 6 ounces canned light tuna (packed in water) with 1 tablespoon reduced-fat mayonnaise. Top one 6" whole wheat flour tortilla* with an unlimited amount of field greens, ¼ cup sliced onion, ¼ cup chopped or sliced tomato, and ½ cup sliced cucumber (or enjoy the cucumber on the side). Add the tuna and wrap tightly.

Water/seltzer/unsweetened iced tea

* Choose whole wheat tortillas with 100 calories or less per tortilla. You may substitute a spinach or sun-dried tomato tortilla.

PM SNACK

Choose any snack from the 100-Calorie Snack List (page 320).

DINNER

1½ cups Extra-Lean Turkey Chili* (page 273)

1 cup sliced cucumber

1 cup sliced red, green, or yellow pepper

Water/seltzer/unsweetened iced tea

* You may substitute any prepared turkey or vegetarian chili with 200 calories or less per 1 cup.

DAY 6

BREAKFAST

Mixed berry and yogurt parfait

Parfait: In a tall parfait glass, alternate layers of mixed berries (using 1 cup sliced strawberries and $\frac{1}{2}$ cup blueberries) with 6 ounces fat-free flavored yogurt.

Tea/coffee

AM SNACK

Choose any snack from the 100-Calorie Snack List (page 320).

LUNCH

Roast beef and Brie on a roll

Sandwich: Spread $\frac{1}{2}$ whole grain sandwich bun* with 1 tablespoon Brie cheese. Top with arugula leaves**, 3 ounces deli-sliced lean roast beef, 1 tomato slice, and 2 teaspoons low-calorie ranch dressing. Eat open faced.

1 cup sliced red, yellow, or green pepper

1 sliced cucumber

Water/seltzer/unsweetened iced tea

* You may substitute $\frac{1}{2}$ of any whole grain roll with 150 calories or less per roll.

** You may substitute any lettuce for the arugula.

PM SNACK

Choose any snack from the 100-Calorie Snack List (page 320).

DINNER

Black Bean and Cheese Burrito

1 frozen black bean and cheese burrito*, heated, topped with:

$\frac{1}{4}$ cup salsa

1 tablespoon fat-free or reduced-fat sour cream

1 cup baby carrots

Water/seltzer/unsweetened iced tea

* Choose frozen burritos with 280 calories or less per burrito.

DAY 7

BREAKFAST

Hard-boiled egg with toasted english muffin and peanut butter

1 hard-boiled (or poached) egg

½ whole wheat English muffin topped with:

2 level teaspoons peanut butter*

Tea/coffee

* You may substitute 1 tablespoon reduced-fat soft cream cheese or 1 ounce fat-free cheese (or ¾ ounce reduced-fat cheese).

AM SNACK

Choose any snack from the 100-Calorie Snack List (page 320).

LUNCH

Spicy Vegetable Roll-Ups with cottage cheese

1 serving Spicy Vegetable Roll-Ups (page 280)

½ cup fat-free or 1% reduced-fat cottage cheese with optional unlimited cinnamon

Water/seltzer/unsweetened iced tea

PM SNACK

Choose any snack from the 100-Calorie Snack List (page 320).

DINNER

1 serving Rosemary Chicken with Grilled Zucchini (page 279)

1 serving Tomato and Green Pepper Salad (page 281)

Water/seltzer/unsweetened iced tea

DAY 8

BREAKFAST

Vanilla-pumpkin breakfast pudding

Pudding: Combine 8 ounces vanilla fat-free yogurt with $1/2$ cup 100% pure canned pumpkin until thoroughly mixed. Sprinkle 1 tablespoon wheat germ on top.

Tea/coffee

AM SNACK

Choose any snack from the 100-Calorie Snack List (page 320).

LUNCH

Hummus garden wrap

Wrap: Spread one 6" whole wheat flour tortilla* with $1/3$ cup hummus (store-bought is fine, any flavor). Top with slices of unpeeled cucumber, 1 loosely packed cup baby spinach leaves, a few pinches of fresh or dried Italian parsley, 2 thin slices of onion, and 8 quartered cherry tomatoes. Roll up and enjoy!

Water/seltzer/unsweetened iced tea

* Choose whole wheat tortillas with 100 calories or less per tortilla.

PM SNACK

Choose any snack from the 100-Calorie Snack List (page 320).

DINNER

Broiled pork tenderloin with baked potato and vegetables

4 ounces lean pork tenderloin, broiled

$1/2$ medium baked potato topped with:

1 tablespoon fat-free or reduced-fat sour cream

1 cup steamed vegetables (broccoli, cauliflower, brussels sprouts, or green beans)

Water/seltzer/unsweetened iced tea

DAY 9

BREAKFAST

Cantaloupe with cottage cheese and slivered almonds

¼ cantaloupe

½ cup fat-free or 1% reduced-fat cottage cheese mixed with:

1 tablespoon slivered almonds and optional cinnamon

Tea/coffee

AM SNACK

Choose any snack from the 100-Calorie Snack List (page 320).

LUNCH

Steamed Chinese food

½ order steamed shrimp (or chicken or tofu) with mixed vegetables

½ cup steamed brown rice

Unlimited low-sodium soy sauce

Chinese mustard (optional)

Water/seltzer/unsweetened iced tea

PM SNACK

Choose any snack from the 100-Calorie Snack List (page 320).

DINNER

Prevention Chicken Burger with sautéed spinach

1 Prevention Chicken Burger* (page 278), no bun

Spinach: Sauté 1 cup spinach (or 1 cup frozen mixed vegetables with 80 calories or less per cup) in 1 teaspoon olive oil and 1 minced clove garlic.

Mixed green salad: Cover a plate with an unlimited amount of romaine lettuce, ½ cup halved cherry tomatoes, and ½ cup chopped cucumber or ½ cup chopped red, green, or yellow pepper. Toss with 2 to 4 tablespoons low-calorie salad dressing.

Water/seltzer/unsweetened iced tea

* You may substitute any prepared turkey, chicken, or veggie burger with 170 calories or less.

DAY 10

BREAKFAST

Instant oatmeal with soy sausage

> 1 packet instant oatmeal* cooked with water, mixed with:
>> Optional cinnamon or nutmeg and sugar substitute
> 1 soy sausage link**

Tea/coffee

* Choose any brand or flavor instant oatmeal with 150 calories or less per packet, preferably a low-sugar variety.

** Choose soy sausage with 40 calories or less per link.

AM SNACK

Choose any snack from the 100-Calorie Snack List (page 320).

LUNCH

English muffin pizza

Pizza: Toast 1 whole wheat English muffin. Top with ¼ cup tomato or marinara sauce* and ¼ cup shredded reduced-fat mozzarella cheese. Bake at 350°F until cheese is melted.

1 cup sliced red, yellow, or green pepper

Water/seltzer/unsweetened iced tea

* Choose sauce with 60 calories or less per ½ cup.

PM SNACK

Choose any snack from the 100-Calorie Snack List (page 320).

DINNER

1½ cups Whole Wheat Penne with Chicken and Broccoli (page 283)

Mixed green salad: Cover a plate with an unlimited amount of romaine lettuce, ½ cup halved cherry tomatoes, and ½ cup chopped cucumber or ½ cup chopped red, green, or yellow pepper. Toss with 2 tablespoons low-calorie salad dressing.

Water/seltzer/unsweetened iced tea

DAY 11

BREAKFAST

Breakfast BLT

BLT: Place 3 slices cooked lean turkey bacon, 2 slices tomato, 1 lettuce leaf, and optional 1 teaspoon reduced-fat mayonnaise on ½ toasted whole grain English muffin.

Tea/coffee

AM SNACK

Choose any snack from the 100-Calorie Snack List (page 320).

LUNCH

Chicken and spinach salad

Salad: Heat a grill or pan to medium high. Coat with cooking spray. Season a 4-ounce chicken breast with salt, pepper, and preferred seasonings and grill until cooked through, 8 to 10 minutes. Transfer to a plate to cool, then slice into strips. Peel and section 1 mandarin orange (or tangerine). Mix chicken and orange with an unlimited amount of raw spinach leaves, 1 tablespoon chopped walnuts, ½ sliced tomato, ¼ chopped or sliced onion, and 2 tablespoons low-calorie salad dressing.

Water/seltzer/unsweetened iced tea

PM SNACK

Choose any snack from the 100-Calorie Snack List (page 320).

DINNER

Grilled bay scallops with vegetables

Scallops: Place 5 ounces bay scallops in a baking dish coated with cooking spray. Drizzle with 2 teaspoons olive oil and add ½ teaspoon dried basil and lemon juice, salt, and pepper to taste. Bake at 350°F for 4 to 5 minutes, until opaque.

1 to 2 cups steamed vegetables*

Water/seltzer/unsweetened iced tea

* If using frozen mixed vegetables, choose those with 80 calories or less per 1 cup. If preparing fresh vegetables, enjoy 2 cups cooked.

DAY 12

BREAKFAST

Sunny-side-up egg on whole grain toast

Egg: Cook 1 whole egg sunny-side up over medium-high heat in a nonstick pan coated with cooking spray.

1 slice whole grain toast* spread with:

1 level tablespoon reduced-fat, soft tub, trans fat–free margarine spread

Tea/coffee

* Choose whole grain bread with 80 calories or less per slice.

AM SNACK

Choose any snack from the 100-Calorie Snack List (page 320).

LUNCH

Roasted vegetable and goat cheese sandwich

Sandwich: Place vegetables (¼ sliced eggplant, ½ cup sliced zucchini, ½ sliced tomato, ½ sliced bell pepper) on a baking sheet coated with cooking spray. Drizzle with 2 teaspoons olive oil. Roast on upper rack of 350°F oven for 20 to 30 minutes. Toast 2 slices reduced-calorie whole grain bread*; spread 1 slice with 1 ounce goat cheese, and layer the roasted vegetables on top. Drizzle with an unlimited amount of balsamic vinegar and top with a second slice of toast spread with optional 1 teaspoon mustard.

Water/seltzer/unsweetened iced tea

* Choose reduced-calorie whole grain bread with 45 calories or less per slice.

PM SNACK

Choose any snack from the 100-Calorie Snack List (page 320).

DINNER

Lean Beef Fajitas (page 276)

Water/seltzer/unsweetened iced tea

DAY 13

BREAKFAST

Whole Grain Mini-Muffin with cottage cheese

1 Whole Grain Mini-Muffin (page 282)

½ cup fat-free or 1% reduced-fat cottage cheese mixed with optional cinnamon

Tea/coffee

AM SNACK

Choose any snack from the 100-Calorie Snack List (page 320).

LUNCH

1 serving Middle Eastern Chicken Salad with Tahini Dressing (page 277)

½ mini whole wheat pita*, toasted

Water/seltzer/unsweetened iced tea

* Choose mini whole wheat pitas with 70 calories or less per pita.

PM SNACK

Choose any snack from the 100-Calorie Snack List (page 320).

DINNER

Grilled fish with wild rice and snow peas

Fish: Season 4 ounces of your favorite fish with 1 teaspoon olive oil and lemon juice, salt, and pepper to taste. Grill until cooked through.

¾ cup cooked wild rice (or brown rice or whole wheat couscous)*

1 cup steamed snow pea pods

Water/seltzer/unsweetened iced tea

* Choose brown rice, wild rice, or whole wheat couscous with 110 calories per ½ cup cooked.

DAY 14

BREAKFAST

Scrambled breakfast wrap

Wrap: Coat a nonstick pan with cooking spray and heat over medium heat. Cook $\frac{1}{2}$ cup chopped or diced mushrooms and onions* until soft. Add $\frac{1}{2}$ cup egg substitute** and 2 tablespoons shredded fat-free cheese (or 1 tablespoon reduced-fat cheese). Scramble until the eggs are cooked and the cheese is melted. Place in the center of 1 warmed 6" whole wheat flour tortilla*** and roll up.

Tea/coffee

* You may substitute $\frac{1}{4}$ cup chopped tomato for the onion.

** You may substitute 3 egg whites.

*** Choose whole wheat tortillas with 100 calories or less per tortilla. You may substitute spinach or sun-dried tomato tortillas.

AM SNACK

Choose any snack from the 100-Calorie Snack List (page 320).

LUNCH

Mexican stuffed baked potato

Potato: Bake 1 medium potato at 350°F until a fork easily pierces it, 45 minutes to 1 hour. Meanwhile, brown 2 ounces lean ground chicken breast over medium-high heat. Slice open the potato, add the cooked chicken, and top with 2 tablespoons shredded fat-free cheese and $\frac{1}{4}$ cup salsa. Bake until the cheese is melted.

Water/seltzer/unsweetened iced tea

PM SNACK

Choose any snack from the 100-Calorie Snack List (page 320).

DINNER

Grilled turkey burger with mixed green salad

Burger: Cook a 5-ounce lean ground turkey patty* (seasoned to taste) under the broiler, on the grill, or in a nonstick pan. Top with 2 tablespoons ketchup, lettuce, and 1 slice tomato.

Salad: Cover a plate with an unlimited amount of romaine lettuce, $\frac{1}{2}$ cup sliced mushrooms, and $\frac{1}{2}$ cup chopped cucumber or $\frac{1}{2}$ cup diced red, green, or yellow pepper. Toss with 2 tablespoons low-calorie salad dressing.

Water/seltzer/unsweetened iced tea

* You may substitute a frozen turkey burger with less than 250 calories.

DAY 1

BREAKFAST

Melon with yogurt, wheat germ, and low-fat granola

$\frac{1}{2}$ cantaloupe

6 ounces fat-free flavored yogurt (or $\frac{1}{2}$ cup fat-free or 1% reduced-fat cottage cheese)
mixed with:

1 teaspoon wheat germ

2 tablespoons low-fat granola cereal

Tea/coffee

AM SNACK

Choose any snack from the 100-Calorie Snack List (page 320).

LUNCH

Open-faced turkey reuben sandwich

Sandwich: Spread up to 2 tablespoons low-calorie Russian dressing onto 2 slices
reduced-calorie whole grain toast.* Top each slice with 2 ounces lean turkey breast (4
ounces total), 1 heaping tablespoon sauerkraut (2 tablespoons total), 1 tomato slice,
optional onion slice, and 1 slice reduced-fat Swiss cheese (about 1 ounce total). Bake in
350°F toaster oven until cheese is melted.

$\frac{1}{2}$ cup red, yellow, or green pepper sticks

Water/seltzer/unsweetened iced tea

* Choose reduced-calorie whole grain bread with 45 calories or less per slice.

PM SNACK

Choose any snack from the 150-Calorie Snack List (page 322).

DINNER

Fish Kebabs with Rice

Fish Kebabs (page 274)

$\frac{1}{2}$ cup steamed brown or wild rice*

1 cup steamed spinach or asparagus

Water/seltzer/unsweetened iced tea

* Choose brown or wild rice with 110 calories or less per $\frac{1}{2}$ cup cooked.

DAY 2

BREAKFAST

Toast with cream cheese, tomato, onion, and lox

    2 slices reduced-calorie whole grain toast* topped with:

        2 level tablespoons reduced-fat soft cream cheese

        2 slices tomato

        Optional sliced onion

        2 ounces lox (smoked salmon)

Tea/coffee

* Choose reduced-calorie whole grain bread with 45 calories or less per slice.

AM SNACK

Choose any snack from the 100-Calorie Snack List (page 320).

LUNCH

Crispy Chicken Tenders with Honey-Dijon Sauce* (page 271)

1 cup sliced red, green, or yellow pepper

Unlimited celery sticks

1 cup red or green grapes

Water/seltzer/unsweetened iced tea

* You may substitute frozen vegetarian soy nuggets with 240 calories or less per serving.

PM SNACK

Choose any snack from the 150-Calorie Snack List (page 322).

DINNER

Eggplant Parmigiana with Edamame

    1 serving Eggplant Parmigiana (page 272)

    1 cup boiled soybeans in the pod, lightly salted

Red, yellow, and green pepper sticks

Water/seltzer/unsweetened iced tea

DAY 3

BREAKFAST

Broccoli and mushroom omelet with turkey bacon and toast

Omelet: Sauté ¹/₂ cup chopped broccoli and ¹/₂ cup sliced (or diced) mushrooms until soft. Add 1 cup whipped egg substitute*, brown on both sides, and fold over.

1 slice turkey bacon

1 slice whole grain toast**, dry

Tea/coffee

* Choose egg substitute with 30 calories or less per ¹/₄ cup.

** Choose whole grain bread with 80 calories or less per slice.

AM SNACK

Choose any snack from the 100-Calorie Snack List (page 320).

LUNCH

Vegetable bean soup with salad

2¹/₂ cups healthy vegetable bean soup*

Salad: Cover a plate with an unlimited amount of romaine lettuce, ¹/₂ cup halved cherry tomatoes, ¹/₂ cup red, green, or yellow pepper, and ¹/₂ cup chopped cucumbers. Toss with 2 tablespoons low-calorie salad dressing.

Water/seltzer/unsweetened iced tea

* Choose canned soup with 125 calories or less per 1 cup.

PM SNACK

Choose any snack from the 150-Calorie Snack List (page 322).

DINNER

Barbecued chicken with spinach and corn on the cob

Chicken: Grill a 5-ounce chicken breast over medium-high heat until cooked through. Top with 2 tablespoons barbecue sauce*.

1 cup steamed spinach

1 medium ear of corn, boiled or grilled, with salt and pepper

Mixed green salad: Cover a plate with an unlimited amount of romaine lettuce, ¹/₂ sliced tomato, and ¹/₂ cup chopped cucumber or ¹/₂ cup chopped red, green, or yellow pepper. Mix with 3 tablespoons low-calorie salad dressing.

Water/seltzer/unsweetened iced tea

* Choose sauce with 50 calories or less per 2 tablespoons.

1,500 **CALORIE PLAN** Phase 2

DAY 4

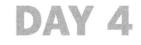

BREAKFAST

Whole grain cereal with nuts and berries

¾ to 1 cup whole grain cereal* topped with:

½ cup fat-free milk

1 tablespoon chopped nuts (almonds, walnuts, and pecans)

½ cup berries

Tea/coffee

* Choose whole grain cereal with 120 calories or less and 3 or more grams of fiber per ¾ to 1 cup.

AM SNACK

Choose any snack from the 100-Calorie Snack List (page 320).

LUNCH

Turkey hot dog with mixed green salad

1 reduced-fat turkey hot dog* with 2 tablespoons sauerkraut, unlimited mustard, and 1 whole wheat hot dog bun**

Salad: Cover a plate with romaine lettuce, ½ cup halved cherry tomatoes, ½ cup chopped bell pepper, ½ cup chopped cucumbers, and ¼ cup chickpeas (rinsed and drained). Toss with 4 tablespoons low-calorie salad dressing.

Water/seltzer/unsweetened iced tea

* Choose turkey hot dogs with 90 calories or less per dog.

** Choose whole wheat buns with 110 calories or less per bun.

PM SNACK

Choose any snack from the 150-Calorie Snack List (page 322).

DINNER

Whole wheat pasta primavera with grilled chicken

Pasta: Cook 2 ounces whole wheat linguine or spaghetti according to package directions (makes 1 cup cooked); drain. Steam 1 cup chopped broccoli (fresh or frozen) and ½ cup sliced mushrooms and add to pasta. Stir in ½ cup tomato or marinara* sauce and top with 1 tablespoon grated Parmesan cheese.

3 ounces grilled chicken breast

Spinach salad: Cover a plate with spinach leaves, sliced cucumbers, and sliced mushrooms. Toss with 2 tablespoons low-calorie salad dressing.

Water/seltzer/unsweetened iced tea

* Choose sauce with 60 calories or less per ½ cup.

DAY 5

BREAKFAST

Berry-Banana Smoothie with scrambled egg whites

1 serving Berry-Banana Smoothie (page 269)

Egg whites: Whip 3 egg whites and scramble in a nonstick pan over medium heat, mixing in 1 ounce shredded fat-free cheese (or ¾ ounce reduced-fat cheese). Season with salt and pepper to taste.

Tea/coffee

AM SNACK

Choose any snack from the 100-Calorie Snack List (page 320).

LUNCH

Garden tuna wrap

Wrap: Combine 6 ounces canned light tuna (packed in water) with 1 tablespoon reduced-fat mayonnaise. Top one 6" whole wheat flour tortilla* with an unlimited amount of field greens, ¼ cup sliced onion, ½ cup sliced cucumber (or enjoy the cucumber on the side), and ¼ cup chopped or sliced tomato. Add the tuna and wrap tightly.

1 cup baby carrots

Water/seltzer/unsweetened iced tea

* Choose whole wheat tortillas with 100 calories or less per tortilla. Or substitute a spinach or sun-dried tomato tortilla.

PM SNACK

Choose any snack from the 150-Calorie Snack List (page 322).

DINNER

1 serving Extra-Lean Turkey Chili* (page 273)

1 cup sliced cucumber

1 cup sliced red, green, or yellow pepper

Water/seltzer/unsweetened iced tea

* You may substitute any prepared turkey or vegetarian chili with 200 calories or less per 1 cup.

1,500 CALORIE PLAN Phase 2

DAY 6

BREAKFAST

Mixed berry and yogurt parfait

Parfait: In a tall parfait glass, alternate layers of mixed berries (using 1 cup sliced strawberries and ½ cup blueberries) with 6 ounces fat-free flavored yogurt. Sprinkle 1 tablespoon wheat germ on top.

Tea/coffee

AM SNACK

Choose any snack from the 100-Calorie Snack List (page 320).

LUNCH

Roast beef and Brie on a roll

Sandwich: Slice 1 whole wheat sandwich bun* in half. Spread 1 tablespoon Brie cheese on the bottom half. Top with arugula leaves**, 3 ounces deli-sliced lean roast beef, 1 small sliced tomato, and 2 teaspoons low-calorie ranch dressing. Cover with the bun top.

1 cup sliced red, yellow, or green pepper

1 sliced cucumber

Water/seltzer/unsweetened iced tea

* You may substitute any whole grain roll with 150 calories or less per roll.

** You may substitute any lettuce for arugula.

PM SNACK

Choose any snack from the 150-Calorie Snack List (page 322).

DINNER

Black bean and cheese burrito with rice

1 frozen black bean and cheese burrito*, heated, topped with:
  ¼ cup salsa
  2 tablespoons fat-free or reduced-fat sour cream
½ cup steamed brown rice**

½ cup baby carrots

Water/seltzer/unsweetened iced tea

* Choose frozen burritos with 280 calories or less per burrito.

** Choose brown rice with 110 calories or less per ½ cup cooked.

DAY 7

BREAKFAST

Hard-boiled egg with toasted english muffin and peanut butter

1 hard-boiled (or poached) egg

½ whole wheat English muffin topped with:

2 level teaspoons peanut butter*

½ cup berries (or ½ grapefruit or orange)

Tea/coffee

* You may substitute 1 tablespoon reduced-fat soft cream cheese or 1 ounce fat-free cheese (or ¾ ounce reduced-fat cheese).

AM SNACK

Choose any snack from the 100-Calorie Snack List (page 320).

LUNCH

Spicy Vegetable Roll-Ups with cottage cheese

1 serving Spicy Vegetable Roll-Ups (page 280)

1 cup fat-free or 1% reduced-fat cottage cheese with optional cinnamon

Water/seltzer/unsweetened iced tea

PM SNACK

Choose any snack from the 150-Calorie Snack List (page 322).

DINNER

Rosemary Chicken with Grilled Zucchini and couscous

1 serving Rosemary Chicken with Grilled Zucchini (page 279)

½ cup whole wheat couscous*

1 serving Tomato and Green Pepper Salad (page 281)

Water/seltzer/unsweetened iced tea

* Choose whole wheat couscous with 110 calories or less per ½ cup cooked.

DAY 8

BREAKFAST

Vanilla-pumpkin breakfast pudding

Pudding: Combine 8 ounces vanilla fat-free yogurt and ½ cup 100% pure canned pumpkin until thoroughly mixed. Sprinkle 1 tablespoon wheat germ on top.

½ sliced banana

Tea/coffee

AM SNACK

Choose any snack from the 100-Calorie Snack List (page 320).

LUNCH

Hummus Garden Wrap

Wrap: Spread one 6" whole wheat flour tortilla* with ½ cup hummus (store-bought is fine, any flavor). Top with 8 thin slices unpeeled cucumber, 1 loosely packed cup baby spinach leaves, a few pinches of fresh or dried Italian parsley, 2 thin slices onion, and 8 quartered cherry tomatoes. Roll up and enjoy!

½ cup baby carrots

Water/seltzer/unsweetened iced tea

* Choose whole wheat tortillas with 100 calories or less.

PM SNACK

Choose any snack from the 150-Calorie Snack List (page 322).

DINNER

Broiled pork tenderloin with baked potato and vegetables

    4 ounces lean pork tenderloin, broiled

    1 medium baked potato topped with:

        1 tablespoon fat-free or reduced-fat sour cream

    1 cup steamed vegetables (broccoli, cauliflower, brussels sprouts, or green beans)

Water/seltzer/unsweetened iced tea

DAY 9

BREAKFAST

Cantaloupe with cottage cheese and slivered almonds

$\frac{1}{2}$ cantaloupe

$\frac{1}{2}$ cup fat-free or 1% reduced-fat cottage cheese mixed with:

Optional cinnamon

1 tablespoon wheat germ

1 tablespoon slivered almonds

Tea/coffee

AM SNACK

Choose any snack from the 100-Calorie Snack List (page 320).

LUNCH

Steamed Chinese food

$\frac{3}{4}$ order of steamed shrimp (or chicken or tofu) with mixed vegetables

$\frac{1}{2}$ cup steamed brown rice

Unlimited low-sodium soy sauce

Optional Chinese mustard

Water/seltzer/unsweetened iced tea

PM SNACK

Choose any snack from the 150-Calorie Snack List (page 322).

DINNER

Prevention Chicken Burger with Fresh Mango Chutney and sautéed spinach

1 Prevention Chicken Burger* (page 278)

1 whole wheat hamburger bun**

1 serving Fresh Mango Chutney (page 275) or $\frac{1}{4}$ cup store-bought plain chutney or mango salsa

Spinach: Sauté 2 to 3 cups spinach (or 1 cup frozen mixed vegetables with 80 calories or less per cup) in 1 teaspoon olive oil and 1 clove minced garlic.

Water/seltzer/unsweetened iced tea

* You may substitute any prepared turkey, chicken, or veggie burger with 170 calories or less.

** Choose whole wheat buns with 150 calories or less per bun.

DAY 10

BREAKFAST

Instant oatmeal with soy sausage

    1 packet instant oatmeal* prepared with water and mixed with:

        Optional cinnamon or nutmeg and sugar substitute

    2 soy sausage links** (or 2 slices lean turkey bacon)

Tea/coffee

* Choose any brand or flavor instant oatmeal with 150 calories or less per packet, preferably a low-sugar variety.

** Choose soy sausage with 40 calories or less per link.

AM SNACK

Choose any snack from the 100-Calorie Snack List (page 320).

LUNCH

English muffin pizza with vegetable salad

    Pizza: Toast 1 whole wheat English muffin. Top with ¼ cup tomato or marinara sauce* and ¼ cup shredded reduced-fat mozzarella cheese. Bake at 350°F until cheese is melted.

    Salad: Cover a plate with an unlimited amount of field greens and fresh vegetables of your choice. Top with 2 tablespoons canned chickpeas (rinsed and drained) and toss with 1 teaspoon olive oil and 1 tablespoon vinegar or fresh lemon juice.

Water/seltzer/unsweetened iced tea

* Choose sauce with 60 calories or less per ½ cup.

PM SNACK

Choose any snack from the 150-Calorie Snack List (page 322).

DINNER

1 serving Whole Wheat Penne with Chicken and Broccoli (page 283)

Mixed green salad: Cover a plate with an unlimited amount of romaine lettuce, ½ cup halved cherry tomatoes, and ½ cup chopped cucumber or ½ cup red, green, or yellow pepper. Toss with 2 tablespoons low-calorie salad dressing.

Water/seltzer/unsweetened iced tea

DAY 11

BREAKFAST

Breakfast BLT

BLT: Place 2 slices cooked lean turkey bacon, 4 slices tomato, 1 lettuce leaf, and optional 1 teaspoon reduced-fat mayonnaise on 1 toasted whole grain English muffin.

Tea/coffee

AM SNACK

Choose any snack from the 100-Calorie Snack List (page 320).

LUNCH

Chicken and Spinach Citrus Salad with Feta Cheese (page 270)

Water/seltzer/unsweetened iced tea

PM SNACK

Choose any snack from the 150-Calorie Snack List (page 322).

DINNER

Grilled bay scallops with baked sweet potato and vegetables

Scallops: Place 5 ounces bay scallops in a baking dish coated with cooking spray. Drizzle with 2 teaspoons olive oil and add $\frac{1}{2}$ teaspoon dried basil and lemon juice, salt, and pepper to taste. Bake at 350°F for 4 to 5 minutes, until opaque.

Sweet potato: Wrap $\frac{1}{2}$ medium (5" long) sweet potato (including skin) in foil and bake at 350°F for 45 minutes to 1 hour, until you can easily pierce with a fork. Season with salt and pepper to taste.

1 to 2 cups steamed vegetables*

Water/seltzer/unsweetened iced tea

* If using frozen mixed vegetables, choose those with 80 calories or less per 1 cup. If preparing fresh vegetables, enjoy 2 cups cooked.

DAY 12

BREAKFAST

Sunny-side-up egg on whole grain toast

Egg: Cook 1 whole egg sunny-side up over medium-high heat in a nonstick pan coated with cooking spray.

1 slice whole grain toast* with:

1 ounce fat-free cheese (or ³⁄₄ ounce reduced-fat cheese)

1 level tablespoon reduced-fat, soft tub, trans fat–free margarine spread

Tea/coffee

* Choose whole grain bread with 80 calories or less per slice.

AM SNACK

Choose any snack from the 100-Calorie Snack List (page 320).

LUNCH

Roasted vegetable and goat cheese sandwich

Sandwich: Place vegetables (¼ sliced eggplant, ½ cup sliced zucchini, ½ sliced tomato, ½ sliced bell pepper) on a baking sheet coated with cooking spray. Drizzle with 2 teaspoons olive oil. Roast on upper rack of 350°F oven for 20 to 30 minutes. Toast 2 slices reduced-calorie whole grain bread*. Spread 1 slice with 1 ounce goat cheese and layer roasted vegetables on top. Drizzle with an unlimited amount of balsamic vinegar and top with a second slice of toast spread with optional 1 teaspoon mustard.

6 ounces fat-free plain or flavored yogurt

Water/seltzer/unsweetened iced tea

* Choose reduced-calorie whole grain bread with 45 calories or less per slice.

PM SNACK

Choose any snack from the 150-Calorie Snack List (page 322).

DINNER

Lean Beef Fajitas (page 276)

Water/seltzer/unsweetened iced tea

DAY 13

BREAKFAST

Whole Grain Mini-Muffin with cottage cheese

1 Whole Grain Mini-Muffin (page 282)

¾ cup fat-free or 1% reduced-fat cottage cheese mixed with optional cinnamon

Tea/coffee

AM SNACK

Choose any snack from the 100-Calorie Snack List (page 320).

LUNCH

1 serving Middle Eastern Chicken Salad with Tahini Dressing (page 277)

1 mini whole wheat pita*, toasted

1 cup baby carrots

Water/seltzer/unsweetened iced tea

* Choose mini whole wheat pitas with 70 calories or less per pita.

PM SNACK

Choose any snack from the 150-Calorie Snack List (page 322).

DINNER

Chilled shrimp cocktail with grilled fish, wild rice, and snow peas

Shrimp: Steam 4 or 5 large shrimp until cooked through; refrigerate until chilled. Serve with 2 tablespoons cocktail sauce and 1 lemon wedge.

Fish: Season 4 ounces of your favorite fish with 1 teaspoon olive oil and lemon juice, salt, and pepper to taste. Grill until cooked through.

¾ cup cooked wild rice (or brown rice or whole wheat couscous)*

1 cup steamed snow pea pods

Water/seltzer/unsweetened iced tea

* Choose brown rice, wild rice, or whole wheat couscous with 110 calories per ½ cup cooked.

DAY 14

BREAKFAST

Scrambled breakfast wrap

Wrap: Coat a nonstick pan with cooking spray and heat over medium-high heat. Cook ½ cup chopped or diced mushrooms and onions and ½ cup chopped broccoli until soft. Add ¾ cup egg substitute and ¼ cup shredded fat-free cheese (or 2 tablespoons reduced-fat cheese). Scramble until eggs are cooked and cheese is melted. Place in the center of 1 warmed 6" whole wheat flour tortilla* and roll up.

Tea/coffee

* Choose whole wheat tortillas with 100 calories or less.

AM SNACK

Choose any snack from the 100-Calorie Snack List (page 320).

LUNCH

Mexican stuffed potato

Potato: Bake 1 medium potato at 350°F until a fork easily pierces it, 45 minutes to 1 hour. Meanwhile, brown 2 ounces lean ground chicken breast over medium-high heat. Slice open the potato, add the cooked chicken, and top with 2 tablespoons shredded fat-free cheese and ¼ cup salsa. Bake until cheese is melted. Top with 2 tablespoons fat-free or reduced-fat sour cream.

1 cup baby carrots and/or red, green, or yellow pepper sticks with salsa

Water/seltzer/unsweetened iced tea

PM SNACK

Choose any snack from the 150-Calorie Snack List (page 322).

DINNER

Grilled turkey burger with Baked French Fries and mixed green salad

Burger: Cook a 5-ounce lean ground turkey patty* (seasoned to taste) under the broiler, on the grill, or in a nonstick pan. Top with 2 tablespoons ketchup, lettuce, and 1 slice tomato.

½ serving Baked French Fries (page 268)

Salad: Cover a plate with an unlimited amount of romaine lettuce, ½ cup sliced mushrooms, and ½ cup chopped cucumber or ½ cup chopped red, green, or yellow pepper. Toss with 2 tablespoons low-calorie salad dressing.

Water/seltzer/unsweetened iced tea

*You may substitute a frozen turkey burger with less than 250 calories.

DAY 1

BREAKFAST

Melon with yogurt, wheat germ, and low-fat granola

½ cantaloupe

6 ounces fat-free flavored yogurt (or ½ cup fat-free or 1% reduced-fat cottage cheese) mixed with:

1 teaspoon wheat germ

¼ cup low-fat granola cereal

Tea/coffee

AM SNACK

Choose any snack from the 150-Calorie Snack List (page 322).

LUNCH

Open-faced turkey Reuben sandwich

Sandwich: Spread up to 3 tablespoons low-calorie Russian dressing on 2 slices reduced-calorie whole grain toast*. Top each slice with 2 ounces lean turkey breast (4 ounces total), 1 heaping tablespoon sauerkraut (2 tablespoons total), 1 tomato slice, optional onion slice, and 1 slice reduced-fat Swiss cheese (about 1 ounce total). Bake in 350°F toaster oven until cheese is melted.

1 cup red, yellow, or green pepper sticks

Water/seltzer/unsweetened iced tea

* Choose reduced-calorie whole grain bread with 45 calories or less per slice.

PM SNACK

Choose any snack from the 200-Calorie Snack List (page 324).

DINNER

Fish Kebabs with Rice

Fish Kebabs (page 274)

¾ cup steamed brown or wild rice*

1 cup steamed spinach or asparagus

Water/seltzer/unsweetened iced tea

* Choose brown or wild rice with 110 calories per ½ cup cooked.

DAY 2

BREAKFAST

Toast with cream cheese, tomato, onion, and lox

    2 slices reduced-calorie whole grain toast* topped with:

        2 level tablespoons reduced-fat soft cream cheese

        2 slices tomato

        Optional sliced onion

        2 ounces lox (smoked salmon)

½ grapefruit

Tea/coffee

* Choose reduced-calorie whole grain bread with 45 calories or less per slice.

AM SNACK

Choose any snack from the 150-Calorie Snack List (page 322).

LUNCH

Crispy Chicken Tenders with Honey-Dijon Sauce

    Crispy Chicken Tenders with Honey-Dijon Sauce* (page 271)

1 cup cooked broccoli or green beans topped with:

    2 tablespoons grated Parmesan cheese

1 cup red or green grapes (or 1 apple, pear, or grapefruit)

Water/seltzer/unsweetened iced tea

* You may substitute frozen vegetarian soy nuggets with 240 calories or less per serving.

PM SNACK

Choose any snack from the 200-Calorie Snack List (page 324).

DINNER

Eggplant Parmigiana with edamame

    1 serving Eggplant Parmigiana (page 272)

    1 cup boiled soybeans in the pod, lightly salted

Mixed green salad: Cover a plate with an unlimited amount of romaine lettuce, ½ cup halved cherry tomatoes, ½ cup chopped red, green, or yellow pepper, and ½ cup chopped cucumber. Toss with 2 to 4 tablespoons low-calorie salad dressing.

Water/seltzer/unsweetened iced tea

DAY 3

BREAKFAST

Broccoli and mushroom omelet with turkey bacon and toast

Omelet: Sauté ½ cup chopped broccoli and ½ cup sliced mushrooms until soft. Add 1 cup egg substitute*, brown, fold, and heat until cooked through.

2 slices cooked lean turkey bacon

1 slice whole grain toast** topped with:

Optional 1 teaspoon reduced-fat, soft tub, trans fat–free margarine spread

Tea/coffee

* Choose egg substitute with 30 calories or less per ¼ cup. Or use 1 egg whipped with 2 egg whites.

** Choose whole grain bread with 80 calories or less per slice.

AM SNACK

Choose any snack from the 150-Calorie Snack List (page 322).

LUNCH

Vegetable bean soup with salad

3 cups healthy vegetable bean soup*

Salad: Cover a plate with an unlimited amount of romaine lettuce, ½ cup halved cherry tomatoes, ½ cup chopped red, green, or yellow pepper, and ½ cup chopped cucumber. Toss with 2 tablespoons low-calorie salad dressing.

Water/seltzer/unsweetened iced tea

* Choose canned soup with 125 calories or less per 1 cup.

PM SNACK

Choose any snack from the 200-Calorie Snack List (page 324).

DINNER

Barbecued chicken with spinach and corn on the cob

Chicken: Grill a 5-ounce skinless boneless chicken breast over medium-high heat until cooked through. Top with 2 tablespoons barbecue sauce*.

1 cup steamed spinach

1 medium ear of corn, boiled or grilled, with salt and pepper

Mixed green salad: Cover a plate with romaine lettuce, ½ sliced tomato, ½ cup chopped cucumber, ½ cup chopped bell pepper, and ½ cup canned chickpeas (rinsed and drained). Toss with 3 tablespoons low-calorie salad dressing.

Water/seltzer/unsweetened iced tea

* Choose sauce with 50 calories or less per 2 tablespoons.

1,800 CALORIE PLAN Phase 2

DAY 4

BREAKFAST

Whole grain cereal with nuts and berries

¾ to 1 cup whole grain cereal* topped with:

½ cup fat-free milk

2 tablespoons chopped nuts (almonds, walnuts, and pecans)

½ cup berries

Tea/coffee

* Choose whole grain cereal with 120 calories or less and 3 or more grams fiber per ¾ to 1 cup.

AM SNACK

Choose any snack from the 150-Calorie Snack List (page 322).

LUNCH

Turkey hot dog with mixed green salad

1 reduced-fat turkey hot dog* with 2 tablespoons sauerkraut, unlimited mustard, and 1 whole wheat hot dog bun**

Salad: Place romaine lettuce on a plate with ½ cup halved cherry tomatoes, ½ cup chopped bell pepper, ½ cup chopped cucumber, and ¼ cup canned chickpeas (rinsed and drained). Toss with 4 tablespoons low-calorie salad dressing.

1 orange (or 1 peach, 1 plum, or ½ grapefruit)

Water/seltzer/unsweetened iced tea

* Choose turkey hot dogs with 90 calories or less per dog.

** Choose whole wheat buns with 110 calories or less per bun.

PM SNACK

Choose any snack from the 200-Calorie Snack List (page 324).

DINNER

Whole wheat pasta primavera with grilled chicken

Pasta: Cook 3 ounces whole wheat pasta according to package directions. Steam 1 cup chopped broccoli and ½ cup sliced mushrooms and add to pasta. Stir in ½ cup tomato or marinara sauce* and top with 1 tablespoon grated Parmesan cheese.

3 ounces grilled chicken breast

Spinach salad: Cover a plate with unlimited spinach leaves, sliced cucumbers, and sliced mushrooms. Toss with 2 tablespoons low-calorie salad dressing.

Water/seltzer/unsweetened iced tea

* Choose sauce with 60 calories or less per ½ cup.

DAY 5

BREAKFAST

Berry-Banana Smoothie with scrambled egg whites and toast

1 serving Berry-Banana Smoothie (page 269)

Egg whites: Whip 3 egg whites and scramble in a nonstick pan over medium heat, mixing in 1 ounce shredded fat-free cheese (or ¾ ounce reduced-fat cheese). Season with salt and pepper to taste.

1 slice reduced-calorie whole grain toast*

Tea/coffee

* Choose reduced-calorie whole grain bread with 45 calories or less per slice.

AM SNACK

Choose any snack from the 150-Calorie Snack List (page 322).

LUNCH

Garden tuna wrap

Wrap: Combine 6 ounces canned light tuna (packed in water) with 1 tablespoon reduced-fat mayonnaise. Top one 6" whole wheat flour tortilla* with an unlimited amount of field greens, ¼ cup sliced onion, ¼ cup chopped or sliced tomato, and ½ cup sliced cucumber (or enjoy the cucumber on the side). Add 1 slice fat-free cheese (or ¾ ounce reduced-fat cheese) and the tuna and wrap tightly.

1 cup baby carrots with:

1 tablespoon low-calorie salad dressing

Water/seltzer/unsweetened iced tea

* Choose whole wheat tortillas with 100 calories or less.

PM SNACK

Choose any snack from the 200-Calorie Snack List (page 324).

DINNER

1 serving Extra-Lean Turkey Chili* (page 273) topped with:

¼ cup shredded fat-free cheese (or 2 tablespoons reduced-fat cheese)

2 tablespoons fat-free or reduced-fat sour cream

Unlimited sliced cucumbers and sliced red, green, or yellow pepper

Water/seltzer/unsweetened iced tea

* You may substitute any prepared turkey or vegetarian chili with 200 calories or less per cup.

DAY 6

BREAKFAST

Mixed berry and yogurt parfait

Parfait: In a tall parfait glass, alternate layers of mixed berries (using 1 cup sliced strawberries and ½ cup blueberries) with 6 ounces fat-free flavored yogurt. Sprinkle 1 to 2 tablespoons wheat germ and 1 tablespoon chopped almonds on top.

Tea/coffee

AM SNACK

Choose any snack from the 150-Calorie Snack List (page 322).

LUNCH

Roast beef and Brie on a roll

Sandwich: Slice 1 whole grain sandwich bun in half. Spread 1 tablespoon Brie cheese on the bottom half. Top with arugula leaves, 3 ounces deli-sliced lean roast beef, 1 tomato slice, and 2 teaspoons low-calorie ranch dressing. Cover with the bun top.

1 cup sliced red, yellow, or green pepper

1 sliced cucumber

½ thinly sliced apple*

Water/seltzer/unsweetened iced tea

* Add the apple to the sandwich or eat on the side.

PM SNACK

Choose any snack from the 200-Calorie Snack List (page 324).

DINNER

Black bean and cheese burrito with rice

1 frozen black bean and cheese burrito*, heated, topped with:
   ½ cup salsa
   2 tablespoons fat-free or reduced-fat sour cream
¾ cup steamed brown rice**

1 cup baby carrots

Water/seltzer/unsweetened iced tea

* Choose frozen burritos with 280 calories or less per burrito.

** Choose brown rice with 110 calories per ½ cup cooked.

DAY 7

BREAKFAST

Hard-boiled egg with toasted english muffin and peanut butter

1 hard-boiled (or poached) egg

½ whole wheat English muffin topped with:

2 level teaspoons peanut butter*

1 cup mixed berries (or 1 banana)

Tea/coffee

* You may substitute 1 tablespoon reduced-fat soft cream cheese or 1 ounce fat-free cheese (or ¾ ounce reduced-fat cheese).

AM SNACK

Choose any snack from the 150-Calorie Snack List (page 322).

LUNCH

Spicy Vegetable Roll-Ups with cottage cheese

1 serving Spicy Vegetable Roll-Ups (page 280)

1 cup fat-free or 1% reduced-fat cottage cheese mixed with optional cinnamon

½ cup fresh blueberries

Water/seltzer/unsweetened iced tea

PM SNACK

Choose any snack from the 200-Calorie Snack List (page 324).

DINNER

Rosemary Chicken with Grilled Zucchini and couscous

1 serving Rosemary Chicken with Grilled Zucchini (page 279)

¾ cup cooked whole wheat couscous*

1 serving Tomato and Green Pepper Salad (page 281) with:

2 tablespoons canned chickpeas (rinsed and drained)

Water/seltzer/unsweetened iced tea

* Choose whole wheat couscous with 110 calories or less per ½ cup cooked.

DAY 8

BREAKFAST

Vanilla-pumpkin breakfast pudding

Pudding: Combine 8 ounces vanilla fat-free yogurt with $\frac{1}{2}$ cup 100% pure canned pumpkin until thoroughly mixed. Mix with:

$\frac{1}{2}$ sliced banana

1 tablespoon chopped walnuts or slivered almonds

1 tablespoon wheat germ

Tea/coffee

AM SNACK

Choose any snack from the 150-Calorie Snack List (page 322).

LUNCH

Hummus garden wrap

Wrap: Spread one 6" whole wheat flour tortilla* with $\frac{1}{2}$ cup hummus (store-bought is fine, any flavor). Top with 8 thin slices unpeeled cucumber, 1 loosely packed cup baby spinach leaves, a few pinches fresh or dried Italian parsley, 2 thin slices onion, and 8 quartered cherry tomatoes. Roll up and enjoy!

$\frac{1}{2}$ cup baby carrots

$\frac{3}{4}$ cup red, purple, or green grapes

Water/seltzer/unsweetened iced tea

* Choose whole wheat tortillas with 100 calories or less per tortilla.

PM SNACK

Choose any snack from the 200-Calorie Snack List (page 324).

DINNER

Broiled pork tenderloin with baked potato and vegetables

5 ounces lean pork tenderloin, broiled

1 medium baked potato topped with:

3 tablespoons fat-free or reduced-fat sour cream

1 cup steamed vegetables (broccoli, cauliflower, brussels sprouts, or green beans)

Water/seltzer/unsweetened iced tea

DAY 9

BREAKFAST

Cantaloupe with cottage cheese and slivered almonds

½ cantaloupe

½ cup fat-free or 1% reduced-fat cottage cheese mixed with:

Optional cinnamon

½ ounce raisins (mini box or 2 tablespoons)

1 tablespoon sliced almonds (or chopped walnuts)

1 tablespoon sunflower seeds (or 2 tablespoons low-fat granola cereal)

Tea/coffee

AM SNACK

Choose any snack from the 150-Calorie Snack List (page 322).

LUNCH

Steamed Chinese food

1 full order steamed shrimp (or chicken or tofu) with mixed vegetables

½ cup steamed brown rice

Unlimited low sodium soy sauce

Chinese mustard (optional)

Water/seltzer/unsweetened iced tea

PM SNACK

Choose any snack from the 200-Calorie Snack List (page 324).

DINNER

Prevention Chicken Burger with Fresh Mango Chutney and sautéed spinach

1 Prevention Chicken Burger (page 278)

1 whole grain hamburger bun*

1 serving Fresh Mango Chutney (page 275)

Spinach: Sauté 2 to 3 cups spinach (or 1 cup frozen mixed vegetables with 80 calories or less per cup) in 1 teaspoon olive oil and 1 clove minced garlic.

Mixed green salad: Cover a plate with an unlimited amount of romaine lettuce, ½ cup halved cherry tomatoes, and ½ cup chopped cucumber or ½ cup chopped red, green, or yellow pepper. Toss with 2 tablespoons low-calorie salad dressing.

Water/seltzer/unsweetened iced tea

* Choose whole wheat buns with 150 calories or less per bun.

DAY 10

BREAKFAST

Instant oatmeal with soy sausage

1 packet instant oatmeal* cooked with water and mixed with:

Optional cinnamon or nutmeg and sugar substitute

4 soy sausage links** (or 4 slices lean turkey bacon)

Tea/coffee

* Choose any brand or flavor instant oatmeal with 150 calories or less per packet, preferably a low-sugar variety.

** Choose soy sausage with 40 calories or less per link.

AM SNACK

Choose any snack from the 150-Calorie Snack List (page 322).

LUNCH

English Muffin pizza with vegetable salad

Pizza: Toast 1 whole wheat English muffin. Top with ¼ cup tomato or marinara sauce* and ¼ cup reduced-fat mozzarella cheese. Bake at 350°F until cheese is melted.

Salad: Cover a plate with an unlimited amount of field greens and fresh vegetables of your choice. Top with ¼ cup canned chickpeas (rinsed and drained) and toss with 2 teaspoons olive oil and 2 to 4 tablespoons vinegar or fresh lemon juice.

Water/seltzer/unsweetened iced tea

* Choose sauce with 60 calories or less per ½ cup.

PM SNACK

Choose any snack from the 200-Calorie Snack List (page 324).

DINNER

2½ cups Whole Wheat Penne with Chicken and Broccoli (page 283)

Mixed green salad: Cover a plate with an unlimited amount of romaine lettuce, ½ cup halved cherry tomatoes, and ½ cup chopped cucumber or ½ cup chopped red, green, or yellow pepper. Toss with 2 tablespoons low-calorie salad dressing.

Water/seltzer/unsweetened iced tea

DAY 11

BREAKFAST

Breakfast BLT

BLT: Place 3 slices lean cooked turkey bacon, 4 or 5 slices tomato, 1 lettuce leaf, and optional 2 teaspoons reduced-fat mayonnaise on 1 toasted whole grain English muffin.

Tea/coffee

AM SNACK

Choose any snack from the 150-Calorie Snack List (page 322).

LUNCH

1 serving Chicken and Spinach Citrus Salad with Feta Cheese (page 270)

1 mini whole wheat pita*

Water/seltzer/unsweetened iced tea

* Choose mini whole wheat pitas with 70 calories or less per pita.

PM SNACK

Choose any snack from the 200-Calorie Snack List (page 324).

DINNER

Grilled bay scallops with baked sweet potato and vegetables

Scallops: Place 5 ounces bay scallops in a baking dish coated with cooking spray. Drizzle with 2 teaspoons olive oil and add $1/2$ teaspoon dried basil and lemon juice, salt, and pepper to taste. Bake at 350°F for 4 to 5 minutes, until opaque.

Sweet potato: Wrap 1 medium (5" long) sweet potato (including skin) in foil and bake at 350°F for 45 minutes to 1 hour, until you can easily pierce it with a fork. Season with salt and pepper to taste.

1 to 2 cups steamed vegetables*

Water/seltzer/unsweetened iced tea

* If using frozen mixed vegetables, choose those with 80 calories or less per 1 cup. If preparing fresh vegetables, enjoy 2 cups cooked.

DAY 12

BREAKFAST

Sunny-side-up egg on whole grain toast

Egg: Cook 1 whole egg sunny-side up over medium-high heat in a nonstick pan coated with cooking spray.

1 slice whole grain toast* with:

1 ounce fat-free cheese (or ¾ ounce reduced-fat cheese)

1 level tablespoon reduced-fat, soft tub, trans fat–free margarine spread

1 cup berries

Tea/coffee

* Choose whole grain bread with 80 calories or less per slice.

AM SNACK

Choose any snack from the 150-Calorie Snack List (page 322).

LUNCH

Roasted vegetable and goat cheese sandwich

Sandwich: Place vegetables (¼ sliced eggplant, ½ cup sliced zucchini, ½ sliced tomato, ½ sliced bell pepper) on a baking sheet coated with cooking spray. Drizzle with 2 teaspoons olive oil. Roast on upper rack of 350°F oven for 20 to 30 minutes. Toast 2 slices reduced-calorie whole grain bread*. Spread 1 slice with 1 ounce goat cheese and layer roasted vegetables on top. Drizzle with an unlimited amount of balsamic vinegar and top with a second slice of toast spread with optional 1 teaspoon mustard.

6 ounces fat-free plain or flavored yogurt mixed with:

2 tablespoons wheat germ (or 1 tablespoon slivered almonds or chopped walnuts)

Water/seltzer/unsweetened iced tea

* Choose reduced-calorie whole grain bread with 45 calories or less per slice.

PM SNACK

Choose any snack from the 200-Calorie Snack List (page 324).

DINNER

Lean Beef Fajitas (page 276)

Water/seltzer/unsweetened iced tea

DAY 13

BREAKFAST

Whole Grain Mini-Muffin with cottage cheese

1 Whole Grain Mini-Muffin (page 282)

1 cup fat-free or 1% reduced-fat cottage cheese mixed with optional cinnamon

Tea/coffee

AM SNACK

Choose any snack from the 150-Calorie Snack List (page 322).

LUNCH

1 serving Middle Eastern Chicken Salad with Tahini Dressing (page 277)

1 regular-size whole wheat pita*, toasted

1 cup baby carrots

Water/seltzer/unsweetened iced tea

* Choose regular whole wheat pitas with 150 calories or less per pita.

PM SNACK

Choose any snack from the 200-Calorie Snack List (page 324).

DINNER

Chilled shrimp cocktail with grilled fish, wild rice, and snow peas

Shrimp: Steam 6 large shrimp until cooked through; refrigerate until chilled. Serve with 3 tablespoons cocktail sauce and 1 lemon wedge.

Fish: Season 6 ounces of your favorite fish with 1 teaspoon olive oil and lemon juice, salt, and pepper to taste. Grill until cooked through.

$3/4$ cup cooked wild rice (or brown rice or whole wheat couscous)

1 cup steamed snow pea pods

Water/seltzer/unsweetened iced tea

* Choose brown rice, wild rice, or whole wheat couscous with 110 calories per $1/2$ cup cooked.

DAY 14

BREAKFAST

Scrambled breakfast wrap

Wrap: Coat a nonstick pan with cooking spray and heat over medium-high heat. Cook ½ cup chopped or diced mushrooms and onions and ½ cup chopped broccoli until soft. Add ¾ cup egg substitute and ¼ cup shredded fat-free cheese (or 2 tablespoons reduced-fat cheese). Scramble until eggs are cooked and cheese is melted. Place in center of 1 warmed 6" whole wheat flour tortilla* and roll up.

1 slice lean Canadian bacon

Tea/coffee

* Choose whole wheat tortillas with 100 calories or less.

AM SNACK

Choose any snack from the 150-Calorie Snack List (page 322).

LUNCH

Mexican stuffed baked potato

Potato: Bake 1 medium potato at 350°F until a fork easily pierces it, 45 minutes to 1 hour. Meanwhile, brown 2 ounces lean ground chicken breast over medium-high heat. Slice open the potato, add the cooked chicken, and top with 3 tablespoons shredded fat-free cheese and ¼ cup salsa. Bake until cheese is melted. Top with 3 tablespoons fat-free or reduced-fat sour cream.

1 cup baby carrots and/or red, green, or yellow pepper sticks with salsa

Water/seltzer/unsweetened iced tea

PM SNACK

Choose any snack from the 200-Calorie Snack List (page 324).

DINNER

Grilled turkey burger with Baked French Fries and mixed green salad

Burger: Cook a 5-ounce lean ground turkey patty (seasoned to taste) under the broiler, on the grill, or in a nonstick pan. Top with 2 tablespoons ketchup, lettuce, and 1 slice tomato.

1 serving Baked French Fries (page 268)

Salad: Cover a plate with an unlimited amount of romaine lettuce, ½ cup mushrooms, and ½ cup chopped cucumber or ½ cup chopped red, green, or yellow pepper. Toss with 2 tablespoons low-calorie salad dressing.

Water/seltzer/unsweetened iced tea

YOUR PHASE 2 EXERCISE ROUTINE AT A GLANCE

The Phase 2 routine shown at a glance in the following pages depicts more advanced exercise movements than the routine you used in Phase 1. You may be ready for this routine today or you may want to hold off for another few weeks or months. If the latter is the case, continue to follow the Phase 1 routine until you physically feel ready for more. Don't beat yourself up over this. If you are working hard, you'll see great results regardless of which routine you follow.

Similarly, you eventually will want to add a fourth day of exercise, taking a day off between sessions. For example, exercise Sunday, Tuesday, Thursday, and Saturday. Add the extra day when you are ready, whether that's today or a few weeks or even a few months from now. Don't push yourself to add it too soon.

WARMUP

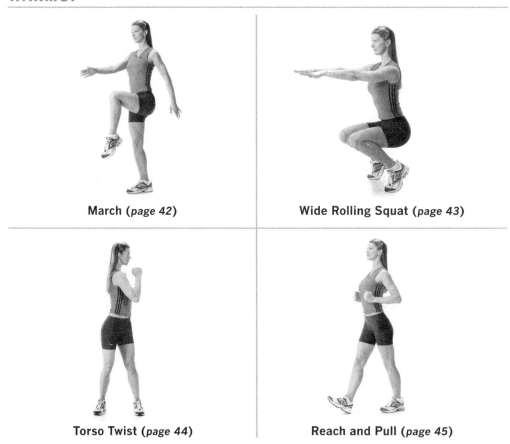

March (*page 42*)

Wide Rolling Squat (*page 43*)

Torso Twist (*page 44*)

Reach and Pull (*page 45*)

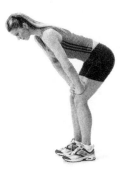

Bend and Round (*page 46*)

ARMS CIRCUIT

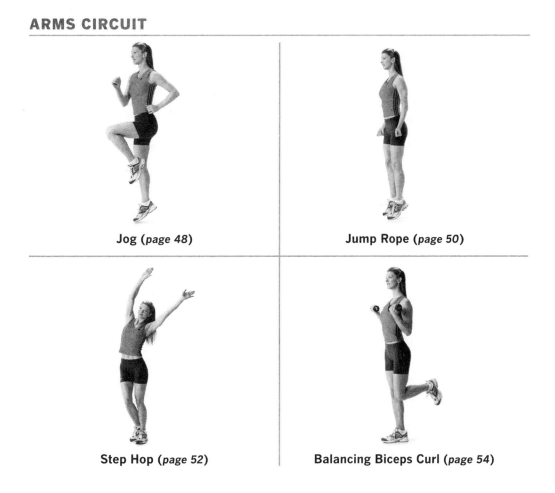

Jog (*page 48*) | **Jump Rope** (*page 50*)

Step Hop (*page 52*) | **Balancing Biceps Curl** (*page 54*)

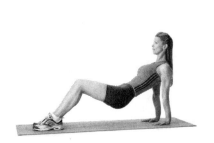

Triceps Dip II (*page 56*)

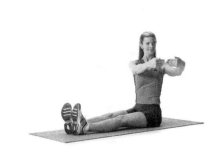

Dandasana Twist (*page 57*)

LEGS AND SHOULDERS CIRCUIT

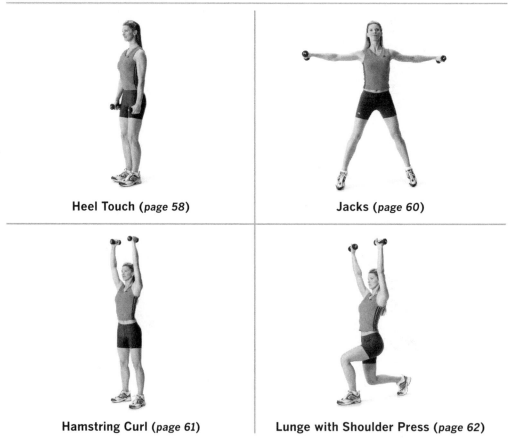

Heel Touch (*page 58*)

Jacks (*page 60*)

Hamstring Curl (*page 61*)

Lunge with Shoulder Press (*page 62*)

LEGS AND SHOULDERS CIRCUIT *continued*

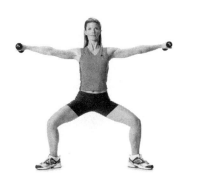

Plié Squat with Shoulder Raise (*page 63*)

Roll Back (*page 64*)

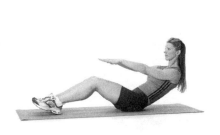

CHEST CIRCUIT

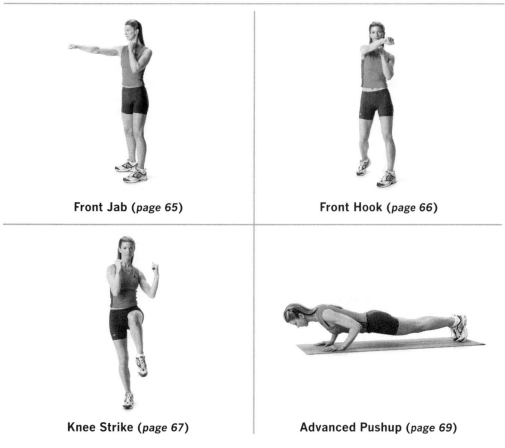

Front Jab (*page 65*)

Front Hook (*page 66*)

Knee Strike (*page 67*)

Advanced Pushup (*page 69*)

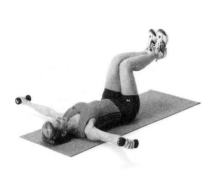

Chest Fly (*page 71*)

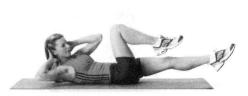

Pilates Bicycle (*page 73*)

BUNS CIRCUIT

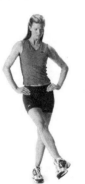

Step Touch with a Soccer Kick (*page 74*)

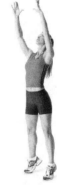

Shoot a Basketball (*page 75*)

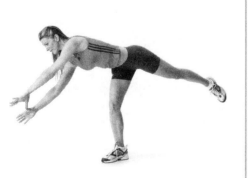

Catch a Football (*page 76*)

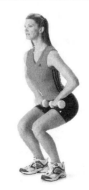

Squat with Leg Lift (*page 78*)

BUNS CIRCUIT *continued*

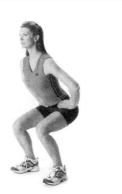

Squat with Front Kick (*page 80*)

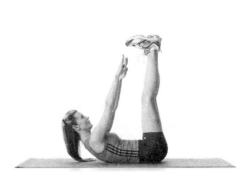

Reverse Curl with Toe Reach (*page 81*)

BACK CIRCUIT

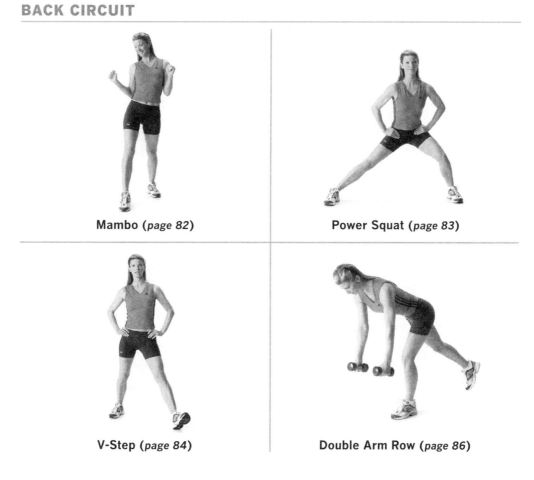

Mambo (*page 82*)

Power Squat (*page 83*)

V-Step (*page 84*)

Double Arm Row (*page 86*)

BACK CIRCUIT *continued*

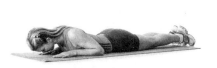

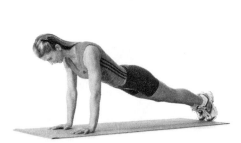

Back Extension (*page 87*)

Body Plank (*page 89*)

COOLDOWN

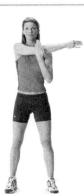

Shoulder Stretch (*page 90*)

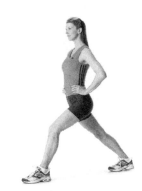

Standing Calf Stretch (*page 91*)

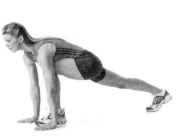

Runner's Stretch (*page 92*)

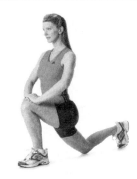

Quad Stretch (*page 93*)

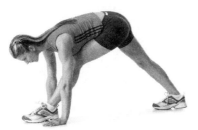

Hamstring Stretch (*page 94***)**

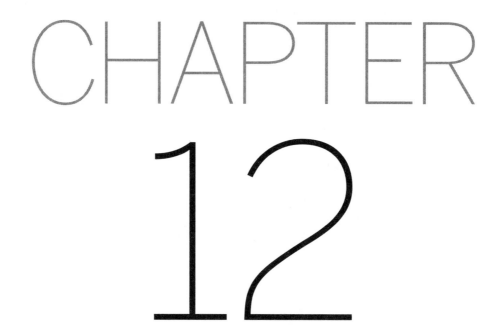

CHAPTER
12

PHASE 2 RECIPES

16 NO-FUSS RECIPES FOR THE WHOLE FAMILY

As with Phase 1, I've tried to keep Phase 2 eating as simple as possible. As you'll see if you flip through the menus, most of the recipes are so short and simple that I've included them in the menu plans. This keeps almost everything in one convenient place, at your fingertips. A few recipes would have taken up too much space in the menus, so I've featured them in the following chapter.

Many of these recipes are my personal favorites. These are the dishes that I like to cook for my family. I hope they become your family favorites as well. Enjoy!

In the following pages, you will find 16 recipes that correspond to the Phase 2 meal plans. Please keep in mind that I did not purposely keep sodium content low in these recipes. If you have a health condition that requires you to watch your sodium intake, please alter them accordingly. I've placed the recipes in alphabetical order to make them easy for you to find and use when you need them. It's very important that you measure your ingredients when making the recipes and eat the appropriate portion size for your individual calorie plan.

BAKED FRENCH FRIES

1 large yam + 1 large russet baking potato (1½ pounds total), peeled and sliced into thin strips

2 tablespoons canola oil

½ teaspoon chili powder

½ teaspoon garlic powder

½ teaspoon ground cumin

½ teaspoon sea salt

1. Preheat the oven to 450°F.

2. Combine the yam and potato, oil, chili powder, garlic powder, and cumin in a bowl and toss well. Arrange in a single layer on a baking sheet. Bake for 25 minutes, turning the fries over with a spatula halfway through, until golden brown. Transfer to a shallow, paper towel–lined bowl and sprinkle with the salt. Serve immediately.

MAKES 4 SERVINGS

PER SERVING: 196 calories, 3 g protein, 31 g carbohydrate, 7 g fat (0 g saturated), 0 mg cholesterol, 302 mg sodium, 3 g fiber

BERRY-BANANA SMOOTHIE

1 cup fat-free milk or low-fat soy milk

1 cup fresh or frozen berries

1 large banana

$\frac{1}{2}$ cup calcium-fortified orange juice

1. In a blender, combine the milk, berries, banana, and orange juice. Process until smooth.

MAKES 2 SERVINGS (1$\frac{1}{4}$ CUPS EACH)

PER SERVING: 146 calories, 6 g protein, 36 g carbohydrate, 0.5 g fat (0 g saturated), 2 mg cholesterol, 55 mg sodium, 4 g fiber

CHICKEN AND SPINACH CITRUS SALAD WITH FETA CHEESE

4 ounces boneless, skinless chicken breast

Salt, freshly ground black pepper, and preferred seasonings to taste

1 mandarin orange or tangerine, peeled and sectioned

Unlimited amount of raw spinach leaves

1 tablespoon chopped walnuts

½ tomato, sliced

¼ onion, chopped

1 ounce crumbled feta cheese

2–4 tablespoons low-calorie salad dressing

1. Heat a grill to medium high. Season the chicken breast with the salt, pepper, and seasonings. Grill until cooked through, about 8 to 10 minutes. Transfer to a plate to cool, then slice into strips. In a large bowl, mix the chicken with the orange, spinach, walnuts, tomato, onion, cheese, and dressing and serve.

MAKES 1 SERVING

PER SERVING: 344 calories, 36 g protein, 25 g carbohydrate, 12.5 g fat (3 g saturated), 76 mg cholesterol, 796 mg sodium, 5 g fiber

CRISPY CHICKEN TENDERS
WITH HONEY-DIJON SAUCE

SAUCE

2 tablespoons plain fat-free yogurt

1 tablespoon fat-free sour cream

1$\frac{1}{2}$ teaspoons Dijon mustard

$\frac{1}{2}$ teaspoon honey

CHICKEN

5 ounces boneless, skinless chicken breast, trimmed and cut into 5 strips

$\frac{1}{4}$ cup crushed cornflakes

$\frac{1}{4}$ teaspoon salt

$\frac{1}{4}$ teaspoon freshly ground black pepper

$\frac{1}{4}$ cup egg substitute, lightly beaten

1 teaspoon olive oil

1. To make the sauce: In a small bowl, combine the yogurt, sour cream, mustard, and honey. Cover and refrigerate.

2. To make the chicken: With a meat mallet, pound the chicken strips to an even thickness. In a shallow bowl, stir together the cornflakes, salt, and pepper. In another shallow bowl, beat the egg substitute and 1 tablespoon water. Dip the chicken strips into the egg mixture and dredge in the cornflake mixture, coating well.

3. Coat a nonstick skillet with cooking spray. Add the oil and heat over medium heat. Add the chicken and cook, turning once, until cooked through and golden brown, about 2 to 3 minutes per side. Serve with the sauce.

MAKES 1 SERVING

PER SERVING: 298 calories, 43 g protein, 17 g carbohydrate, 6.5 g fat (1 g saturated), 84 mg cholesterol, 477 mg sodium, 0 g fiber

EGGPLANT PARMIGIANA

1 large egg, beaten

¼ teaspoon freshly ground black pepper

⅛ teaspoon garlic salt

½ cup dried whole wheat bread crumbs

½ large eggplant, cut into ¼"-thick slices

1 tablespoon olive oil

¾ cup marinara sauce

¼ teaspoon crushed red pepper flakes

½ jar (13 ounces) roasted sweet red peppers, drained

1 cup shredded reduced-fat mozzarella cheese

2 tablespoons grated Parmesan cheese

1. Preheat the oven to 325°F.

2. In a shallow bowl, combine the egg, black pepper, and garlic salt. Place the bread crumbs in another shallow bowl. Dip the eggplant slices in the egg mixture, then dredge in the bread crumbs.

3. Heat the oil in a large nonstick skillet over medium-high heat. Lightly coat the eggplant slices with cooking spray. In batches, add the eggplant to the skillet and cook, turning once, until browned, about 40 minutes.

4. Spread ¼ cup of the sauce on the bottom of a 13" x 9" baking dish. Top with the eggplant slices, remaining sauce, red pepper flakes, and red peppers. Sprinkle with the mozzarella and Parmesan. Bake until cooked through and the cheese is browned, about 40 minutes.

MAKES 4 SERVINGS

PER SERVING: 176 calories, 28 g protein, 10 g carbohydrate, 2 g fat (0.5 g saturated), 66 mg cholesterol, 307 mg sodium, 2 g fiber

EXTRA-LEAN TURKEY CHILI

2 pounds extra-lean ground turkey breast

1 can (12 ounces) crushed tomatoes (without paste)

$\frac{1}{2}$ onion, diced

2 tablespoons chili powder

2 teaspoons garlic powder

1 teaspoon paprika

1 teaspoon ground cumin

1 teaspoon dried oregano

1 teaspoon freshly ground black pepper

$\frac{1}{2}$ teaspoon ground red pepper (or more for hotter chili)

2 teaspoons all-purpose flour

1 can (15 ounces) red kidney beans, rinsed and drained

1. Brown the turkey in a nonstick skillet over medium-high heat, stirring to break up the meat. Drain off any fat. Add $1\frac{1}{2}$ cups water and the tomatoes, onion, chili powder, garlic powder, paprika, cumin, oregano, black pepper, and red pepper and mix thoroughly.

2. Cover and simmer for 25 to 30 minutes, stirring every 10 minutes. Stir in the flour and cook, stirring, for 2 minutes. Add the beans and mix well. Simmer, uncovered, for 20 minutes.

MAKES 4 SERVINGS (2 CUPS EACH)

PER SERVING: 397 calories, 60 g protein, 30 g carbohydrate, 4 g fat (1 g saturated), 90 mg cholesterol, 600 mg sodium, 11 g fiber

FISH KEBABS

½ onion, sliced

1 bell pepper, sliced

4 ounces tilapia, salmon, or black cod, cut into chunks

8 cherry tomatoes

2 teaspoons olive oil

Salt and freshly ground black pepper to taste

1. Coat a nonstick baking sheet with cooking spray. Soak 2 wooden skewers in water for about 30 minutes. Place the onion and pepper in a shallow dish with a little water. Cover with a paper towel and microwave for 1 minute or until soft.

2. Preheat the oven to 350°F. Alternate threading the cooked vegetables, fish, and tomatoes onto the skewers. Place on the coated baking sheet, drizzle with the oil, and season with the salt and pepper. Place on the upper rack of the oven and bake for 15 to 20 minutes, until the vegetables are tender and the fish is cooked through.

MAKES 1 SERVING

PER SERVING: 259 calories, 26 g protein, 16 g carbohydrate, 11.5 g fat (2 g saturated), 57 mg cholesterol, 71 mg sodium, 4 g fiber

FRESH MANGO CHUTNEY

3 cups chopped ripe mangos (3 to 4 mangos)

1/2 cup chopped yellow onion

1/4 cup apple cider vinegar

1/4 cup raisins

1/4 cup packed brown sugar

1 tablespoon finely chopped or grated fresh ginger

1 1/4 teaspoons minced garlic

1 teaspoon finely chopped fresh serrano or jalapeño chile pepper, stems and seeds removed (wear plastic gloves when handling)

1 teaspoon garam masala (Indian spice mixture)*

1 teaspoon finely grated lemon peel

2 tablespoons lemon juice

1 tablespoon finely grated orange peel

1/2 cup orange juice

1. Combine the mangos, onion, vinegar, raisins, brown sugar, ginger, garlic, chile pepper, garam masala, lemon peel, lemon juice, orange peel, and orange juice in a saucepan and bring to a simmer. Cook until softened, 10 to 12 minutes.

2. Pour the mixture through a sieve set over a bowl. Spoon the solids into a large bowl and set aside. Pour the liquid back into the saucepan and cook over high heat, stirring constantly, until reduced to a syrup, about 6 minutes.

3. Fold the syrup into the solids and let cool to room temperature. Store the chutney in an airtight container in the refrigerator for up to 1 month.

MAKES 12 SERVINGS (1/4 CUP EACH)

PER SERVING: 64 calories, 1 g protein, 17 g carbohydrate, 1 g fat (0 g saturated), 0 mg cholesterol, 5 mg sodium, 1 g fiber

*If garam masala is unavailable, substitute a mixture of the following: 1/4 teaspoon ground cardamom, 1/4 teaspoon ground cinnamon, 1/8 teaspoon ground black pepper, 1/8 teaspoon coriander, and 1/8 teaspoon cumin.

LEAN BEEF FAJITAS

5 ounces lean sirloin, trimmed of fat

Salt, freshly ground black pepper, and other preferred seasonings to taste

1 teaspoon olive oil

1 bell pepper, sliced

1 onion, sliced

2 (6-inch) whole wheat tortillas

2 tablespoons salsa

2 tablespoons fat-free or reduced-fat sour cream

Dash of Tabasco (optional)

1. Season the beef with the salt, black pepper, and other seasonings and cook to desired tenderness. Slice into thin strips. Coat a nonstick pan with cooking spray, add the oil, and heat over medium-high heat. Add the pepper, onion, and additional seasoning if desired. Cook until soft. Add the beef and vegetables to the warmed tortillas. Roll up and top with the salsa, sour cream, and Tabasco (if using).

MAKES 1 SERVING

PER SERVING: 552 calories, 39 g protein, 59 g carbohydrate, 17 g fat (3.5 g saturated), 70 mg cholesterol, 686 mg sodium, 10 g fiber

Variation: You may substitute shrimp, chicken, or tofu for the steak in this recipe.

MIDDLE EASTERN CHICKEN SALAD
WITH TAHINI DRESSING

CHICKEN SALAD

2 boneless, skinless chicken breasts (4 ounces each)

1 can (15 ounces) chickpeas, rinsed and drained

3 medium ripe tomatoes, chopped

2 stalks celery, chopped

1/4 cup chopped fresh parsley

DRESSING

1/2 cup plain fat-free yogurt

3 tablespoons tahini (sesame paste)

1 tablespoon lemon juice

1 clove garlic, minced

1 teaspoon ground cumin

1/2 teaspoon kosher salt

1/4 teaspoon ground red pepper

1. To make the chicken salad: Place the chicken in a steamer, cover, and gently steam over simmering water until juicy and just cooked through, 8 to 10 minutes (or grill or boil the chicken). Transfer to a plate to cool. Cut or tear the cooled chicken into bite-size pieces and place in a large bowl. Add the chickpeas, tomatoes, celery, and parsley.

2. To make the dressing: Whisk the yogurt, tahini, lemon juice, garlic, cumin, salt, and pepper in a small bowl until smooth.

3. Just before serving, pour the dressing over the chicken mixture and toss gently to combine.

MAKES 4 SERVINGS

PER SERVING: 267 calories, 21 g protein, 27 g carbohydrate, 9 g fat (1 g saturated), 32 mg cholesterol, 695 mg sodium, 6 g fiber

PREVENTION CHICKEN BURGERS

  1 pound lean ground chicken breast

  1 cup fresh whole wheat bread crumbs

  $^1/_2$ cup chopped red bell pepper

  $^1/_4$ cup chopped green bell pepper

  $^1/_4$ cup chopped red onion

  $^1/_4$ cup chopped celery

  2 tablespoons chopped fresh parsley

  1 tablespoon low-sodium soy sauce

  1 clove garlic, minced

  $^1/_2$ teaspoon dried thyme

  Freshly ground black pepper to taste

1. Preheat the oven to 350°F. Grease a baking sheet.

2. In a large bowl, mix the chicken, bread crumbs, red and green peppers, onion, celery, parsley, soy sauce, garlic, thyme, and black pepper just until combined. Divide the mixture into 4 equal portions and shape into patties.

3. Place the patties on the prepared baking sheet. Bake, turning once, until a thermometer inserted in the center registers 170°F, 25 to 30 minutes.

MAKES 4 SERVINGS

PER SERVING: 170 calories, 28 g protein, 9 g carbohydrate, 2 g fat (0 g saturated), 65 mg cholesterol, 270 mg sodium, 2 g fiber

Variation: If you prefer, cook the patties in 1 to 2 teaspoons canola oil for 8 to 10 minutes per side. You may also use lean ground turkey instead of chicken.

ROSEMARY CHICKEN WITH GRILLED ZUCCHINI

2 tablespoons olive oil

1/4 cup lemon juice

1 tablespoon minced garlic

Kosher salt

Freshly ground black pepper

4 boneless, skinless chicken breasts (1¼ pounds)

2 medium zucchini, sliced lengthwise into 1/4"- to 1/2"-thick pieces

8 (3"–4") sprigs rosemary + additional for garnish

1. Preheat the grill to medium high (350° to 400°F).

2. In a small bowl, gently whisk the oil, lemon juice, and garlic and add salt and pepper to taste. Transfer to a 1-gallon zipper-seal bag. Add the chicken and turn to coat. Gently press the air from the bag and close. Place in a large shallow bowl and refrigerate for 20 minutes to 1 hour.

3. Season the zucchini slices with 1/8 teaspoon salt and 1/8 teaspoon pepper. Remove the chicken from the marinade. Thoroughly coat the zucchini and chicken with cooking spray. Place half of the rosemary sprigs directly on the grill and lay the chicken on top. Place the remaining rosemary on the chicken. Place the zucchini on the grill next to the chicken and rosemary. Grill the chicken, turning once, until a thermometer inserted in the thickest portion registers 160°F and the juices run clear, about 5 to 6 minutes per side. Grill the zucchini, turning once, until tender, about 10 minutes.

4. Arrange equal amounts of the chicken and zucchini on 4 plates. Garnish with rosemary sprigs and serve immediately.

MAKES 4 SERVINGS

PER SERVING: 242 calories, 34 g protein, 6 g carbohydrate, 8 g fat (1 g saturated), 82 mg cholesterol, 164 mg sodium, 2 g fiber

SPICY VEGETABLE ROLL-UPS

½ cup chickpea flour*

6 tablespoons cold water, or more if needed

1½ tablespoons olive oil

½ beaten egg or 2 tablespoons egg substitute

2 pinches of salt

2 pinches of ground black pepper

¼ small onion, finely chopped

½ medium zucchini, finely chopped

½ large head cauliflower, divided into florets and finely chopped

½ teaspoon minced fresh ginger

Pinch of ground cumin

Pinch of crushed red pepper flakes

1 tablespoon tomato sauce

½ scallion, thinly sliced

1. Place the flour in a bowl and gradually whisk in the water to make a smooth, thin batter; add more water if needed. Whisk in 1 tablespoon of the oil, the egg or egg substitute, 1 pinch of salt, and 1 pinch of black pepper.

2. Coat an 8" nonstick skillet with cooking spray and heat over medium heat. Pour 1½ tablespoons batter into the skillet and quickly tilt the skillet to coat the bottom. Cook until the bottom is nicely browned, about 1 minute. Turn the pancake with a spatula and cook 30 to 45 seconds longer (it will look spotty on the bottom). Slide the pancake onto a plate and cover with foil. Repeat with cooking spray and the remaining batter to make 8 pancakes total.

3. Heat the remaining ½ tablespoon oil in another skillet over medium heat. Stir in the onion, zucchini, cauliflower, ginger, cumin, and red pepper flakes. Cover and cook, stirring occasionally, for 3 minutes. Stir in the tomato sauce, cover, and cook until the vegetables are tender and the liquid is evaporated, 10 to 15 minutes. Stir in the scallion, the remaining pinch of salt, and the remaining pinch of pepper.

4. Place a pancake on a plate, attractive side down. Spoon about ¼ cup of the vegetable mixture in a line one-third of the way from one edge and roll up the pancake. Repeat with the remaining pancakes and vegetables.

MAKES 4 SERVINGS (2 ROLL-UPS EACH)

PER SERVING: 50 calories, 2 g protein, 4 g carbohydrate, 3 g fat (0 g saturated), 15 mg cholesterol, 55 mg sodium, 1 g fiber

*Chickpea flour is available in most natural food stores.

TOMATO AND GREEN PEPPER SALAD

3 large green bell peppers, seeded and cut into strips

2 medium tomatoes, diced

2 tablespoons olive oil

1 teaspoon lemon juice

2 cloves garlic, minced

Salt and freshly ground black pepper to taste

Shredded arugula or other lettuce

1. Place the bell peppers and tomatoes in a medium bowl. Toss with the oil, lemon juice, garlic, salt, black pepper, and arugula.

MAKES 4 SERVINGS

PER SERVING: 120 calories, 3 g protein, 11 g carbohydrate, 8 g fat (1 g saturated), 0 mg cholesterol, 20 mg sodium, 4 g fiber

WHOLE GRAIN MINI-MUFFINS

¾ cup 1% reduced-fat milk

⅓ cup wheat germ oil*

3 tablespoons frozen orange juice concentrate, thawed

1 tablespoon grated orange peel

1 egg

2¼ cups whole grain pastry flour

⅓ cup + 1 tablespoon sugar

1 tablespoon baking powder

¼ teaspoon salt

½ cup + 3 tablespoons finely chopped almonds

1. Preheat the oven to 400°F. Coat a 24-cup mini-muffin pan with cooking spray or line with paper liners.

2. Mix the milk, oil, orange juice concentrate, orange peel, and egg in a large bowl. Add the flour, ⅓ cup sugar, and the baking powder and salt. Stir until just combined; do not overmix (the batter should be lumpy). Stir in ½ cup almonds. Divide the batter evenly among the prepared muffin cups and sprinkle with the remaining 1 tablespoon sugar and 3 tablespoons almonds.

3. Bake for 20 to 25 minutes or until golden. Remove the muffins from the pan and cool on a rack.

MAKES 24 MUFFINS

PER SERVING: 65 calories, 2 g protein, 8 g carbohydrate, 3 g fat (0.5 g saturated), 6 mg cholesterol, 61 mg sodium, 1 g fiber

*Wheat germ oil is available in most health food stores. You may substitute canola oil.

WHOLE WHEAT PENNE
WITH CHICKEN AND BROCCOLI

1/4 cup extra-virgin olive oil

1/2 large onion, chopped

4 cloves garlic, minced

1 pound skinless, boneless chicken breasts, cut into 1" cubes

8 cups broccoli florets

1 package (16 ounces) whole wheat penne pasta

2 tablespoons grated Romano cheese

Freshly ground black pepper to taste

1. Bring a large pot of salted water to a rolling boil over high heat.

2. Meanwhile, heat the oil in a medium saucepan over medium heat. Add the onion and garlic and sauté until translucent, being careful not to brown. Add the chicken and cook, stirring, until cooked through. Remove from the heat.

3. Add the broccoli to the boiling water and cook until crisp-tender, about 4 minutes. With a slotted spoon or skimmer, transfer to the saucepan with the chicken. Return the saucepan to medium heat and cook until the broccoli is completely broken down but still green.

4. Return the pot of water to a boil and add the pasta. Cook according to package directions until al dente. Drain, reserving 1 cup cooking water. Add the pasta and water to the broccoli mixture. Toss to mix, add the cheese, and toss again. Serve on individual plates, topped with the black pepper.

MAKES 8 SERVINGS (ABOUT 2 CUPS EACH)

PER SERVING: 378 calories, 23 g protein, 51 g carbohydrate, 9 g fat (1.5 g saturated), 34 mg cholesterol, 231 mg sodium, 8 g fiber

CHAPTER

13

PLATEAU POINTERS

WHAT TO DO IF THE SCALE STALLS

Everyone reaches a plateau from time to time. It's part of the natural process of losing weight. Don't panic. Naturally, you will feel frustrated. That's to be expected, but don't allow your frustration to derail all of your good efforts. Never let a plateau throw you into overeating.

As I mentioned in Chapter 5, your progress may start and stop many times before you reach your final destination. A temporary plateau of up to three weeks may simply be your body adjusting to your new lower weight. Or it can be caused by muscle replacing fat. Muscle is both more compact than and heavier than fat. If you were sedentary when you began 3-2-1 and are now following the 3-2-1 fitness plan consistently, an increase in muscle and other types of lean body mass may cause your weight loss to slow from time to time, even as you continue to shrink your fat cells.

Temporary plateaus may also stem from very slow weight loss. You may still be losing weight, perhaps a fraction of a pound a week. It just may take as long as three weeks for these fractions to add up to a full pound that you can notice and celebrate. Finally, you may be retaining water or even be constipated, both of which can mask fat loss.

To make sure you have hit a true plateau—where no amount of dietary diligence for no amount of time will cause your weight to budge—consider other indicators of your success. How do your clothes fit? Are they roomier? What about your measurements? Are you still losing inches? Have you had your body fat tested lately? Has the percentage improved? If you feel as if you look better, you probably do look better.

Trust your instincts. If your clothing size, measurements, and other indicators are still moving in the right direction, ignore the scale and continue to do what you've been doing so well. Be positive and proud of your accomplishments, and eventually the weight loss will continue. If you're eating smart and exercising regularly, your weight will probably drop in due time. Quite often, I've found that the body must adjust, losing weight and then maintaining for a while. After a few weeks at the same weight, you may very well happily find that your weight goes down again.

If, after four weeks, your weight still doesn't budge, consider whether you are at your appropriate weight. Make sure the long-term goal you set for yourself is realistic. Trying to reduce your weight beyond your body's natural comfort zone (what weight loss experts refer to as your *set weight*) will only result in frustration.

If you're convinced that you've set a realistic long-term goal for yourself, then read on to learn about many factors that tend to hinder weight loss, along with what to do about them.

WHAT'S CAUSING YOUR PLATEAU?

To get past the plateau, you need to figure out what's causing it. Are you sticking with the 3-2-1 plan diligently, putting in the recommended workouts and following the meal plan recommendations without fail? If the answer is yes to all of the above, then you probably hit a plateau simply because your metabolism has slowed. As you lose weight and become smaller, your body naturally burns fewer calories. Simply put, it takes more calories to power a larger body than a smaller one. In this case, skip the rest of this section and go directly to "What to Do about It."

On the other hand, if you are not quite sure you are following 3-2-1 as well as you could, consider going back to the daily food log that you kept for the first few days of the plan. This written record will help you to see in black and white whether you've begun to stray. The truth of the matter is that most people are less regimented with their food intake after their initial weight loss. Use your log to record not only what you eat but also how much and how often you exercise. Keep tabs on how you feel when you eat, particularly when you find yourself going off the plan.

Keep your log for a week and then look it over. You may be struggling because your portion sizes have crept up or your workouts have decreased in intensity or frequency. When you look at your log, look for sneaky extracurricular sources of calories in the form of additional condiments or salad dressings (or nibbles off your child's or spouse's plate). Check to see whether you are eating the prescribed meals in the right portions.

Are you pouring too much cereal into your bowl or dishing yourself too much rice? Did you skip any exercise sessions? Did you overeat at any meals? Did you double a treat? Did you reach for extra snacks?

Don't use this information to beat yourself up. Rather, use it to spot patterns and solve problems. For instance, you might notice that you tend to snack at night, starting with your daily treat but continuing to eat more. Or you may find that you eat a lot of unconscious calories, taking little nibbles here and there. What is your most difficult food time? Is it in the evening after dinner or in the afternoon? Whenever it is, that may be the best time to eat a snack or your treat if you are not doing so already.

In the following pages, you will find advice for solving the problems that your log will probably uncover.

WHAT TO DO ABOUT IT

If you have found that you have stuck to the 3-2-1 plan eating with precision, and you are putting in at least 30 minutes of exercise everyday, it's time to change your routine. To start losing again, you need to work even more diligently. Consider the following options.

- **Switch to a lower-calorie meal plan.** If you are following the 1,500- or 1,800-calorie plan, consider switching to one of the lower-calorie plans.

- **Add more exercise.** If you are doing 3-2-1 workouts three times a week for 30 minutes a day, move up to four times a week. If you are already working out four times a week, try doubling one of your workouts, so you are exercising for an hour on one of your four days. Add other forms of cardio, such as power walking. Try adding an extra 10 minutes of cardio to your daily routine to burn 50 to 100 more calories.

- **Mix things up.** Vary your food and exercise. Sometimes your body just needs a change of scenery. Look through a cookbook for tasty recipes and try new physical activities.

- **Remove all starchy carbohydrates from dinner.** No pasta, rice, bread, potatoes, corn, peas, or quinoa. Instead, load up on plain (no-fat-added) nonstarchy vegetables like broccoli, carrots, peppers, spinach, cauliflower, zucchini, and lettuce. These veggies provide much fewer calories but can really fill you up.

ADDITIONAL REASONS
YOUR WEIGHT LOSS MAY STALL

In the following pages, you will find some common problems that prevented some of my clients from initially losing all the weight they wanted. You'll also find the strategies that these clients used to turn things around—and get their weight moving in the right direction.

Do You Eat When You're under Stress?

You may find that you can follow 3-2-1 *most of the time*, except for certain times when you are under stress or feeling sad, depressed, anxious, or some other negative emotion. Know that many people turn to food to soothe negative emotions. The key is finding another outlet for your stress and negative emotions. Consider the following alternatives.

Chew sugarless gum. You'll reduce stress and satisfy your urge to chew without consuming excess calories.

Squeeze a stress ball. It will keep your hands busy, preventing you from using them to insert food into your mouth. Squeeze your ball over and over until you calm down. If you don't have a ball, consider another way to occupy your hands. Drum them on a table or jiggle the loose change in your pocket.

Write about what's bothering you. Keep a journal, using it to be your own therapist on paper. Whenever you find that you want to soothe your emotions with food, write about what's bothering you. Use the power of the pen (or even keep a journal on your computer if you find it easier to type) to release pent-up emotions. You may find that writing also allows you to take a step back and solve the problem that is causing the negative emotions in the first place. Quite often, once you have finished putting pen to paper, your craving for food will have diminished.

Talk to a friend. As with writing in a journal, talking to a friend can help you solve the problems that are making you feel bad in the first place. Promise yourself that before you turn to food, you will first call a friend. By the end of the conversation, you may feel better, and your urge to eat may have passed.

Create a three-food interference list. If you frequently eat large quantities of food in response to certain moods, think of three low-calorie foods that might satisfy your mood in lieu of your typically high-calorie comfort food. For instance, you might choose two large handfuls of baby carrots, a small container of light yogurt, or an apple. Promise yourself that next time, you will turn to the three foods on your list *before* you turn to the cake, cookies, mashed potatoes, pasta, breakfast cereal, peanut butter, or ice cream. I like to call this *food interference*—and it's been very helpful for many of my clients. As you eat the carrots, yogurt, or apple, an important thing will happen. Time will elapse, and hopefully the urge to feed your emotion will begin to subside. You'll also fill up on your three healthy foods. And most important, you'll be able to gain control of both your mood and your eating before you turn to the high-calorie fare.

Do You Eat When You're Bored?

If you find that you turn to food when you are at loose ends, you will need to find nonfood ways to entertain yourself. Take some time now to create a list of activities that might help fill the time until your next urge to eat or overeat has passed. You might try any of the following.

- Go for a walk
- Knit
- Update photo albums or scrapbooks
- Clean out your closets or your purse
- Do housework
- Give yourself a manicure or pedicure
- Surf the Internet
- Run errands
- Call a friend
- Make upcoming appointments (doctor, dentist, hair, etc.)
- Schedule playdates for your kids
- Listen to favorite music

Come up with a list of activities that work for you. Many of my clients have found that polishing their nails really helps to eliminate boredom-induced eating. You won't want to ruin the polish by eating, and by the time it dries, you will have moved on to something else.

Are You Nibbling?

It's amazing how much extra food we can munch on without realizing it. Not long ago, I counseled a stay-at-home mom, Jill, who told me that for the most part, she was following her meal plan to a T, yet her weight was going in the opposite direction. I began asking her some questions about her eating habits, and soon it was clear to me that Jill was a nibbler. She admitted to eating a nibble here and there—the last bite of her kid's mac and cheese, a handful of Cheerios, and so on. She didn't think these nibbles amounted to much, but I wasn't as convinced. I asked her to carry a zipper-seal bag around with her for one day. "Every time you feel tempted to nibble, I want you to place what you would have sampled into the bag instead of eating it. Then, at the end of the day, bring me the bag so we can see just how much or how little these nibbles are affecting your weight."

She carried the bag around with her. When she brought it back to me, we both had a good laugh. Just one day of potential nibbles had completely filled her bag! When I analyzed the calorie content of the food in the bag, it was about 1,000 calories. No wonder she was gaining rather than losing!

Jill found the bag experiment very useful. It was a nice reality check and encouraged her to be more mindful with her food grabs.

In addition to trying this experiment, you might also benefit from the following tips.

Keep a food log. Write down everything you eat—especially the little nibbles—until you get grazing under control.

Slow your pace. Eat *slowly* and taste your food. You'll feel more satisfied after eating and be less likely to nibble leftovers from a family member's plate.

Eat meals without multitasking. For example, don't eat while watching television, checking e-mails, or talking on the phone. This will ensure that you eat consciously rather than unconsciously.

Do You Lose Control at Night?

As I mentioned earlier, a large number of my overweight clients tend to overeat at night. These nighttime munchers generally put away more calories in the form of post dinner snacks than they eat for dinner. In fact, they can sometimes consume more than half of their daily calories in the evening. Does this sound familiar?

Although 3-2-1 eating will help you break out of this eating pattern, you may need a few additional strategies to put night eating behind you for good.

Consider whether you would be better off eating your treat right before bed. Many of the night eaters that I've counseled have found that they can more easily put a lid on night eating if they have something to look forward to. So rather than have your treat right after dinner, save it for right before bed. Eat it, brush your teeth, and get right into bed.

Try this for a week and see if it works for you. If you still have problems, then you may need to make a no-eating rule at nighttime. For you, any nighttime eating may open a Pandora's box that you don't yet have the mental strength to close. In this case, after dinner, drink herbal or decaf tea to put closure on the meal. Brush and floss your teeth.

Find noneating activities to occupy yourself in the evening. You might tape your favorite soaps or sitcoms during the day so you can watch them at night or keep a large library of DVDs on hand to watch. If you like to read, always have a new book or magazine on deck to pick up as soon as you finish your old one. If you live with others, consider playing cards, board games, dominos, or other activities that keep both your hands and mind busy. Or you can always surf the Web and answer e-mails.

Also take steps to binge-proof your house. On this plan, you have the opportunity for a portion-controlled serving of any food every day. If you tend to lose control with certain foods, however, get them out of your house. Seriously. That way, they can't call your name at night.

Finally, every time you feel the urge to eat, remind yourself over and over again how great you will feel in the morning if you don't.

Do You Stray a Lot Whenever You Stray a Little?

I've counseled many clients who initially had an all-or-nothing mindset about dieting. They felt as if they either were following their meal plan perfectly or that they had completely blown it and might as well give up. For these clients, there was no middle ground. One extra chip at lunch led to overeating and cheating for the rest of the day, week, month, or even season. Eventually, they would start fresh and recommit to losing weight, but they abandoned their efforts so frequently that their weight loss was minimal at best.

Alice was a perfect example. During her first appointment, I asked Alice to recommit to her food plan any time she strayed from it in order to keep her all-or-nothing thinking in check. No indiscretion—no matter how big—could be used as an excuse to give up on her plan. Alice agreed to put it into practice. When she came back for her next appointment, she explained that she was able to go a few days without abandoning her weight loss plan, but whenever she had a bad day, she gave up on eating well.

We devised the following solution. Whenever Alice felt she was having a bad day, she had to write down everything she had eaten as well as a strategy to rectify her indiscretions. To take things a step further, she had to e-mail this list and strategy to a close friend and then call her to talk it over. The end result? Alice would gain an important reality check and slow down. Instead of telling herself, "I've blown it. I might as well eat what I want for the rest of the day," Alice's written notes and telephone conference with her friend helped her to see that she really had not destroyed the whole day. In fact, she was able to see that—in most cases—she could undo the damage by taking an extra walk or eating somewhat less at her next meal.

In addition to trying the food-log technique, read the following whenever you realize that you've slipped up. Use these truths to halt the negative thinking spiral.

- Think about what a friend would do if she had just eaten the same thing. Have any of your thin friends gained 10 pounds just by eating a couple of cookies or a slice of cake?

- You can recover from this—and may still even lose weight. Put a stop to it now and move on.

- It's only when you turn a small indulgence into a full-fledged food orgy that you gain weight rather than lose it.

- Nothing you ate today is so bad that you should go off the plan altogether.

- Stop eating and get back on track—now.

Are You Skimping on 3-2-1 Exercise or Still Being Sedentary?

As I've mentioned before, your 3-2-1 fitness plan does much more than burn off excess calories. It also helps you to better stick with your 3-2-1 meal plan. If you've lost some weight and then hit a plateau, starting your exercise plan will help you to get past that plateau.

To motivate yourself to exercise, remind yourself of the benefits. Not only does it help you to burn calories, but it also keeps your metabolism from dipping. It improves your body shape. Face it, there are some things diet can do and some it can't. Only exercise can firm up flab. It reduces your idle time, which will help you to refrain from eating when bored or at loose ends. It improves your self-esteem so that you remain confident in your ability to stick with 3-2-1 eating. Finally, it improves your health, preventing countless diseases.

So if you are not already doing it, get started. Follow these additional tips to motivate yourself to start and stick with 3-2-1 exercise.

• **Set small, short-term exercise goals.** If you are completely sedentary, your first goal may be to get through one 3-2-1 circuit, then two, and then three. Eventually, your goal will be to get through the entire routine without stopping. Then you can make it your goal to incorporate some of the more challenging movements. Each time you reach a small goal, you will grow more confident in your fitness abilities.

• **Plan exercise into your day.** Take a look at your calendar. When can you fit in your 3-2-1 workouts? Would you rather exercise in the morning or at night? Many of my clients found that they fit in exercise by getting up earlier each morning and doing it first thing. Some studies show that exercisers who work out in the morning are 50 percent more likely to stick with it.

• **Log your workouts.** Writing down what you did is a great way to give yourself a pat on the back. Your exercise log should be a great source of pride. Whenever your motivation is lagging, open your log and use your past accomplishments to encourage you.

KEEP TRYING, KEEP LOSING, KEEP IT OFF

No matter what your reasons for hitting your plateau, you can get through this. If you have a lot of weight to lose, know that you may, from time to time, need to return to this chapter to solve various problems that stand in your way.

The good news is that no problem is too big for you. As long as you remain optimistic and creative, you can do what it takes to move the scale in the right direction—and to keep it there once you reach your goal. As long as you follow the plan, nothing—nothing!—can keep you from changing your body for the better.

3·2·1
SUCCESS STORY
Debbi McCullock

Age: 41
Accomplishment: Lost 7 pounds in four weeks

Q: How did you gain the excess weight?

A: I have been married for 24 years and am a busy mom of four kids, ages 5 to 24, and one precious daughter-in-law. I gained 60 pounds with each of my pregnancies, and that never really came off for good. I am also a licensed minister and a full-time family nurse practitioner. So needless to say, I'm busy. I know how to help people; I help people every day and tell them how to take care of their health and where to find the strength to change their lives. So knowledge about what to do is not my problem. My issues with weight loss have been my busy life and problems with sustaining motivation.

Q: What weight loss programs have you tried in the past?

A: I have lost weight taking diet pills. With pills, I felt horrible, but I was thin. I have also tried-low carb and low-calorie diets, as well as the cabbage soup diet. They all worked in the short term, but then I would give up. I have gone to Weight Watchers with some success, but eventually, it didn't fit into my schedule. Like everyone else, I usually gained back whatever I lost . . . plus interest.

Q: What changes have you noticed in your health?

A: I now have lots of energy! I feel like the Energizer bunny on the days I exercise—I get twice the amount of stuff done because I just keep going . . . and going . . . and going.

Q: What changes have you noticed in your psychological health?

A: I am really happy. It feels wonderful to be doing something good for myself!

Q: What do you think of the exercise on the plan?

A: The 3-2-1 workout is great. I love the circuits, and I love that I could do it from the start, even though I had not exercised in a long time. The exercise is perfect—enough, but not too much.

Q: Overall, what has your experience been with 3-2-1?

A: I love the program! Thank you!

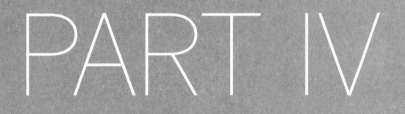

PART IV

Phase 3

CHAPTER
14

PHASE 3 NUTRITION

HOW TO EAT TO KEEP OFF THE WEIGHT

Congratulations on reaching your goal! Bravo—give yourself a pat on the back. You really do deserve it.

You've worked hard to lose the weight and should feel proud of your accomplishment. Be aware, however, that maintaining weight loss is where many of my clients struggle.

I can tell you this: You can do it. You will do it. I know because you have everything you need to maintain your weight loss right here in your hands. You've already proven that you have the motivation and willpower to stick to a weight loss program, and now you need the same motivation, willpower, and stamina for maintenance. People just like you succeed at maintenance every day, month, and year. I know this from reading the results from the National Weight Control Registry—a study of thousands of dieters who have lost 30 pounds or more and who keep it off for more than a year. That's right—it's a study of *thousands* of successful dieters. Keeping off the weight is not impossible. You can do this.

To keep off the weight, you must keep up the effort. Weight maintenance is a lifelong project and a way of living—and as you now know, the rewards are well worth it. As long as you are willing to accept that fact, you will do wonderfully. Now for some fantastic news: The longer you maintain your weight loss, the easier it gets. Studies done on hundreds of successful dieters show that over time, you'll eventually be able to pay less attention to and put less effort into keeping off the weight. For now, however, make keeping it off your number one priority.

3·2·1 TIP

You may have heard that you should weigh yourself only once a week to avoid becoming preoccupied with the scale. That's definitely true as you lose weight, when so many factors can affect your weight from day to day, and any small gain can cause motivation to wane. To maintain your loss, however, daily weighing may be the way to go. Based on results form thousands of people who lost weight, researchers have determined that dieters are more likely to maintain their weight loss if they weigh themselves daily. Frequent weigh-ins can help you to keep tabs on any small gains and to respond immediately if they surpass the 5-pound mark.

WHAT IS MAINTENANCE?

During maintenance, expect to go up and down a few pounds over and over again. Face it, you're human. You go out to eat. You take vacations. You go to social functions during the holidays. You can't expect yourself to hold steady at one number. Small weight fluctuations are normal and expected. Be aware of them and keep them under control, but don't get frustrated and beat yourself up when they happen.

The key is to catch more significant weight gains early, before a minor setback has turned into a weight gain that will take significant time and effort to rectify, affecting your confidence. Use 5 pounds as your red flag. That's when it's time to do something about it in a committed and serious way. It's also time to examine what caused you to gain that much weight, so you can fix the problem and avoid having to work yourself back down to your maintenance weight in the future.

If you gain back 5 pounds or more, do the following.

1. Return to the meal plan you followed during the weight loss phase (or a lower-calorie meal plan if you are currently following a Phase 2 meal plan to maintain).
2. Increase your exercise time, possibly by doubling up on your 3-2-1 circuits or by adding more cardio.
3. If you continually yo-yo, losing 5 or more pounds, gaining 5 or more pounds, then losing again, go back to using a food log (described on page 100). Consider logging your exercise as well. Use the logs to uncover problems. Perhaps your portion sizes have crept up. Perhaps you are cutting more workout sessions shorter than you realize. Perhaps little nibbles are beginning

to add up. Try to learn from the experience. Maybe you need to eat out less often or plan to complete your 3-2-1 fitness routine in the morning, when you have more time.

4. Keep at it and never give up. If you don't nip it in the bud, 5 pounds may turn into 10, 10 pounds into 20, and so on and so on. Don't go there.

HOW TO EAT TO KEEP OFF THE WEIGHT

I wish I could give you a formula that would help you to determine the number of calories you need to eat to keep off the weight. Unfortunately, I can't. Everyone's body responds somewhat differently to weight loss. Some people experience a drop in metabolism as they lose weight. Others experience little to no metabolic slowdown because they've substantially increased their muscle mass. The right amount of food for one woman who weighs 140 pounds may be wildly different from the right amount of food for another woman at the same weight.

I can't nail down a firm number for you, but I can provide you with a rough idea. To keep off the weight, you will need to use one of the following three strategies.

Strategy 1: Eat a bit more than you did to lose the weight. Many women can consume up to 200 more daily calories once they reach their goal. This prevents them from continuing to lose weight beyond their goal. So if you were following the 1,500-calorie plan, you may be able to bump your calorie intake up to 1,700 (see instructions on increasing calories on page 302).

Strategy 2: Eat the same as you did to lose weight. Some dieters reach their goal weight and automatically plateau. To keep off the weight, these dieters have three choices.

1. Follow Phase 2 eating permanently (for the most part).
2. Eat more, but add about 20 minutes of daily exercise.
3. Eat a bit more and keep exercise the same. Be prepared to gain a few pounds and accept yourself at a slightly higher weight than you originally planned.

Strategy 3: Eat less. As you age, your metabolism typically slows, and as your body shrinks in size, it can slow even more. You may have succeeded at losing weight while following the 1,800-calorie plan. However, as you get older (and smaller!), you may find that you gain weight on 1,800 daily calories, and you need to switch to the 1,500-calorie plan to hold the line. The beauty is that 3-2-1 allows you to treat yourself every day. Thus, even if you must continually stay on a version of the food plan to keep off the weight, the 3-2-1 system makes lifelong weight management painless and possible.

■

How do you know which of the three strategies to follow? Trial and error. Start with strategy 1—eating more. Monitor your body closely, using the scale and/or your measurements or clothing fit for feedback. Try to stay within 2 to 3 pounds of your current weight. If your weight or measurements continually creep upward, you're eating too much to maintain your current weight, so move on to strategy 2. Begin following the same calorie plan you used in Phase 2 (or add 20 minutes of extra cardio daily). Keep monitoring your weight. If strategy 2 doesn't work, move on to strategy 3.

HOW TO ADD CALORIES

Okay, so you're starting with strategy 1, eating a bit more. How do you modify Phase 2 eating to allow for up to 200 more daily calories? First, don't forget to use the scale as your guide. Step on the scale once a week or as often as once a day (please, no more than that). This is your project. I can give you a rough idea of how much to eat, but only you can determine the right number of calories for your body.

In the following pages, you'll find three ways to bump up your food intake. Pick an option that feels right to you. To prevent any sudden increases in weight, transition to 3-2-1 maintenance eating very slowly. Start with the smallest change (one treat splurge in a given week, one meal off, or one extra portion of food a day) and increase from there.

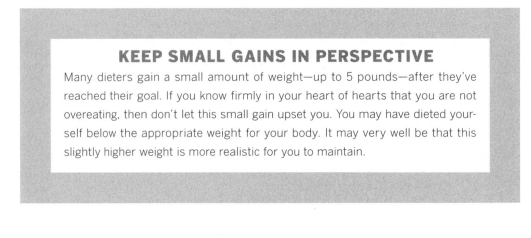

KEEP SMALL GAINS IN PERSPECTIVE

Many dieters gain a small amount of weight—up to 5 pounds—after they've reached their goal. If you know firmly in your heart of hearts that you are not overeating, then don't let this small gain upset you. You may have dieted yourself below the appropriate weight for your body. It may very well be that this slightly higher weight is more realistic for you to maintain.

OPTION 1:
INCREASE THE AMOUNT OF FOOD YOU EAT EVERY DAY

Works best for: People who prefer to eat a greater daily volume of healthy food.

How to do it: Eat the following nonstarchy vegetables in unlimited amounts: asparagus, beets, broccoli, brussels sprouts, cabbage, carrots, cauliflower, celery, cucumbers, eggplant, green beans, greens (collard, mustard, and turnip), kale, kohlrabi, leeks, lettuce, mushrooms, okra, onions, pea pods, peppers (red, yellow, and green), radishes, rutabaga, spinach, sugar snap peas, Swiss chard, tomatoes, water chestnuts, or zucchini.

In addition to rounding out each meal with more veggies, give yourself one or two extra portions of food each day from the categories below. For example, an additional apple and ½ cup brown rice would total two extra portions. Start with one extra portion of food each day for the first week, and if your weight remains stable, increase to two extra portions each day. Use this guide for increasing your portions accordingly.

- **Fruit:** One portion equals 1½ cups whole strawberries, 1 cup berries, 1 cup cubed melon, 1 cup pineapple, ½ cup unsweetened applesauce, 2 tablespoons raisins, ¼ cantaloupe, ½ grapefruit, ½ pomegranate, ½ mango, 1 medium apple, 1 kiwi, 1 nectarine, 1 orange, 1 peach, 1 medium pear, 1 medium watermelon wedge, 2 clementines, 2 figs, 2 persimmons, 2 small plums, 2 tangerines, 4 apricots, 12 large cherries, or 20 grapes.

- **Protein:** One portion equals 2 ounces of lean poultry, lean meat, or fish or 1 whole egg or 4 egg whites.

- **High-quality starch:** One portion equals 1 slice whole wheat bread, 2 slices reduced-calorie bread, 1 small whole wheat pita bread (70 calories), ½ regular whole wheat pita bread, ½ whole grain English muffin, ½ cup cooked brown or wild rice, ½ cup cooked whole wheat pasta, ½ medium baked white potato, ½ medium baked sweet potato, ¾ cup whole grain breakfast cereal (120 calories or less), ½ cup dry plain oatmeal, ½ cup peas, ½ cup corn, ½ cup kidney beans, ½ cup chickpeas, ½ cup acorn or butternut squash.

- **Fats and oils:** One portion equals 1 to 2 teaspoons olive oil, 1 tablespoon regular salad dressing (or 2 to 4 tablespoons low-calorie dressing), 1 tablespoon regular cream cheese (or 2 tablespoons light cream cheese), 1 to 2 tablespoons guacamole, 1 tablespoon regular mayonnaise (or 1 to 2 tablespoons reduced-fat mayonnaise), 1 tablespoon soft tub, trans fat–free margarine (or 2 tablespoons light version), 1 to 2 tablespoons chopped nuts, or 1 level tablespoon peanut butter.

OPTION 2:
FOLLOW YOUR PHASE 2 MEAL PLANS MOST OF THE TIME, BUT TAKE 1 OR 2 MEALS OFF EACH WEEK FOR A SPLURGE

Works best for: People who want the flexibility to eat a favorite meal once or twice each week and are otherwise willing to follow their Phase 2 meal plans the rest of the week.

How to do it: Plan to enjoy a meal that you've been missing while following the 3-2-1 food plan. Maybe it's chicken parmigiana with pasta or maybe a few slices of thin-crust pizza—or maybe your friend is having a dinner party, and you have no control over what she is serving. Whatever the case, you've earned it—enjoy! Just remember these few things: Eat an appropriate portion and do *not* let this turn into a binge. Don't automatically hit the bread basket beforehand or indulge in dessert when dinner is through. Be selective and carefully decide exactly how you will splurge. Do you really love bread? Then have it. If, on the other hand, you're not married to it, skip the bread appetizer. Do you really love mashed potatoes? Great. If not, order the baked potato. During your splurge, eat slowly, enjoying every bite.

If you choose this option, watch your weight carefully. If you are unable to keep your splurge meal from becoming a binge, options 1 and 3 may be a better fit for you as you maintain your healthy goal weight.

3-2-1 **TIP** If you can maintain your weight loss only by strictly following your Phase 2 meal plan, use the following strategy to occasionally indulge in larger portions of your favorite treats. Rather than having a treat from the Treat Lists every day, omit your daily treats most days to bank up some treat calories. Then splurge two or three times a week on a larger-than-usual treat portion.

OPTION 3:
INCREASE THE SIZE OF YOUR TREAT ONCE OR TWICE A WEEK

Works best for: People who absolutely love dessert and other treats and who don't necessarily need to increase the portion sizes of real food at each meal or care about splurging on an entire dinner.

How to do it: Many, many treats do not fit into the Treat Lists starting on page 314. The large slice of pie or cake from your favorite coffee shop or restaurant usually weighs in with over 500 calories. That's more than I'd like you to budget for your treat *every* day, but it's fine to splurge up to two times a week. Use your treat splurge on sweet desserts if you prefer, but you can also use it to splurge on other high-calorie, high-fat foods, such as an occasional side order of french fries, fried onion rings, or wings. Budget for up to 500 calories for your treat splurge. Use the list below as a rough guide, but you certainly do not have to stick with these options. Get a calorie-counting guide or ask the wait staff for the calorie amounts of treats you'd like to order.

- 1 slice chocolate layer cake
- 1 slice carrot cake with cream cheese frosting
- 1 small hot fudge sundae (made with 1 scoop premium ice cream, 1 tablespoon hot fudge, a squirt of whipped cream, and a cherry)
- A plate of chips and guacamole that you share with friends
- 1 margarita
- 1 piña colada

3·2·1
SUCCESS STORY

LeAnn Loche

Age: 37
Accomplishment: Lost 9 pounds, 1½ inches off her waist, 1 inch off her hips, and 1 inch off each thigh in seven weeks.

Q: How did you gain the excess weight?

A: I didn't always struggle with my weight. When I was first married, I weighed 130 pounds. After a few years that included two moves and two children born 10 months apart by C-section, I started gaining weight. At first, I blamed the weight on having children. Now my youngest is 14, so that excuse is long gone.

Q: How does this weight loss plan compare to others you have tried?

A: I have tried and failed on many plans before because I always felt deprived of certain foods. I don't feel that way on this plan. I have never eaten so much on a weight loss plan as I do on 3-2-1. I have always been a snacker, and eating three meals, two snacks, and a treat really satisfies that need.

Q: What changes have you noticed in your physical health?

A: I have noticed a huge difference in my energy level, especially since I am now eating breakfast on a daily basis. Walking on my treadmill is getting easier every day, and I can increase my speed and incline each week. I have also found that my balance has improved since I started the program.

Q: What changes have you noticed in your psychological health?

A: Well, I was taking antidepressants when I started the program and I'm not now, so that says a lot. I have seen a big difference in my mood and the way I feel about myself. I feel a definite change in the way my clothes fit. I am finding that I wear things now that I haven't been able to wear for at least a year. I feel confident that I will continue to my goal, no matter how long it takes.

Q: What do you think of the exercise?

A: I have never been a big exercise fan because I always felt as if I had to spend two to three hours a day exercising to see results. The 3-2-1 workout has been great for me because the segments are both short and effective. I thought there was no way I could do six-minute segments and actually get a good workout but I was completely wrong. I felt muscles the next day that I didn't realize were there!

Q: How do the regular meals affect your success?

A: The regular meals make all the difference in the world. In the past, I ate breakfast very rarely. I would snack a little in the morning, eat lunch, and then snack even more in the afternoon. I never felt satisfied. Now, I am much more aware of what I put in my mouth and *why* I am eating it.

Q: Overall, what is your experience with 3-2-1?

A: I had a wonderful experience with the program, and I continue to have great success. I am working really hard to keep on track and trying to exercise every day. I know the weight did not come on overnight, and it's going to take hard work and time to get it all off, but I am ready for the challenge. I want to do this for myself and accomplish this weight loss to make my family proud.

CHAPTER

15

PHASE 3 FITNESS

HOW TO EXERCISE TO KEEP OFF THE WEIGHT

I hope you've come to love 3-2-1 fitness. Exercising to 3-2-1 is an inspiring, fun, and effective way to work out. To keep off the weight, know that maintaining your exercise routine is just as important as maintaining your new eating habits. Countless studies show that people who exercise are more successful at maintaining weight loss than people who try to slay slim with calorie control alone. If you do the same 3-2-1 circuits in the same order session after session, week after week and month after month, you will probably become bored. If you allow the boredom to persist, you'll eventually skip a session, then another, and then another. Before you know it, you'll be right back where you started.

What to do? Don't allow your 3-2-1 routine to go stale. You can continue to exercise the 3-2-1 way for the rest of your life without ever losing interest. To do so, you need to occasionally freshen up your routine by changing your exercise schedule, the order of your circuits, the weight you lift, and the individual exercises that you complete. This chapter will tell you everything you need to know to stay motivated as you maintain your weight loss.

YOUR 3-2-1 SCHEDULE

You began your 3-2-1 journey by completing three 3-2-1 routines a week, for a total of 90 weekly minutes of exercise. During your weight loss journey, you may have—as the program recommends—added to that amount of exercise, working out to 3-2-1 circuits four times a week. To keep off the weight, you must maintain your effort. So if you are working out three times a week, stick with it. If you're working out four times a week, keep it up!

Regular exercise burns calories as well as preserves muscle mass, which in turn keeps your metabolism humming along as you age. Even with the best exercise program, however, your metabolism will slow with age. As your metabolism slows, you have two options to prevent weight gain. You can either eat less or exercise more (or a combination of both). To add more exercise, consider any of the following options.

• If you are currently working out three days a week, add another 3-2-1 session to your routine. Take a day off between sessions. For example, exercise Sunday, Tuesday, Thursday, and Saturday for one week. The following week, do your 3-2-1 sessions on Monday, Wednesday, and Friday, then start again on Sunday.

• Double one or more of your 3-2-1 sessions. Do your 3-2-1 routine twice, for a total of 60 minutes. This can burn up to 500 calories per session. Or add additional cardio to your week, fitting it in during your days off from 3-2-1. Go for a power walk. Take a bike ride. Swim in a pool. Walk on the treadmill. Choose a cardio option that you love and look forward to completing.

• Add additional spontaneous exercise to each day. If you work in an office building, walk up a flight of stairs a couple of times a day. If you are a full-time mom, play actively with your kids (ride bikes together, get up on the playground equipment with them, take nature walks and hikes).

KEEP YOUR ROUTINE FRESH

As I mentioned before, doing the same routine over and over again gets boring. Not only do you lose interest mentally, but your muscles may also adapt to the repetitive motion, causing you to burn fewer calories per workout. The more unfamiliar your exercise routine, the harder your body must work, and consequently the more calories you burn. So keep changing it up!

You can modify your routine in a number of ways. Below you will find some options. Use the ones that work best for you.

Increase your resistance. Once your 3-2-1 routine begins to feel easy, increase the weight you use. In other words, if you are currently using 5- and 8-pound weights, increase to 8 pounds and 10 or 12 pounds. Each increase in resistance will challenge your muscles a little more. The more you challenge your muscles, the stronger they become, which in turn speeds your metabolism while toning your body.

Keep tabs on your intensity. Don't allow yourself to simply go through the motions. Consider purchasing a heart rate monitor to help you to continually challenge yourself. Try to stay within a specific training zone of 60 to 75 percent of your maximum heart rate. (See page 38 for information on determining your training zone.) After each circuit, glance at your heart rate reading to make sure you are in your zone. If you're below your zone, use that as incentive to pick up the pace.

Change the order of the circuits. Go ahead and mix up your circuits, doing them in a slightly different order each time you work out. Do the routine backward. Work your chest first on one day, your arms first the next, and so on.

Include new cardio options. For each circuit, try new cardio moves. Mix in traditional cardio moves like jumping rope, jacks, and other moves. Have fun and ignite your energy with music you love (anything goes, from Led Zeppelin's greatest hits to the soundtrack of *A Chorus Line*). Think back to high school gym class sessions or previous sports training. Shuffles, bounding, grapevines—anything is fair game as long as it boosts your heart rate. If you have a treadmill, stationary bike, elliptical machine, or other cardio exercise equipment, you can use it. Just make sure you set it so you can quickly hop on and go. You don't want to waste some of your 3 minutes punching instructions into your machine to get it to move.

To freshen up the cardio segments of your 3-2-1 circuits, consider the following ideas.

Jumping rope

Doing jumping jacks

Skipping around the room

Doing grapevines

Doing step touches and other traditional "aerobics" dance movements

Jogging or marching in place

Mountain climbing (Remember elementary school gym class? With your hands and feet on the floor, jog your feet forward and back as if you were climbing a mountain)

Dancing to your favorite music

Shuffling from left to right and right to left (as if you were dribbling a basketball)

Jogging up and down the bottom step of a staircase

Dancing like the Rockettes

Mix in new strength and abdominal moves. Learn different ways to work your major muscle groups. Go to www.prevention.com for new ideas on strengthening your butt, abs, chest, and much more. Gather exercise moves from your favorite videos and DVDs. Consult a personal trainer for ideas. As long as you keep an open mind and continually seek out new ways to move your body, you will never get bored.

Below you'll find additional strengthening options. Go to www.exrx.net/Lists/Directory.html to see videos and detailed instructions for most of the following suggested exercises.

Arms: Hammer curl, preacher curl, concentration curl, seated or standing triceps extension, lying triceps extension, triceps kick back

Shoulders: Front raise, military/shoulder press, Arnold press, upright row, lateral raise, rear deltoid row

Legs: Squat, plié squat, lunge, rear lunge, side lunge, single leg squat, split squat, step up, walking lunge

Chest: Bench press, incline bench press, pushup (hands close, medium, or wide distance), chest fly, pull over

Buns: Squat, lunge, step up, dead lift, side leg lift, hydrant, bridge

Back (upper and lower): Bent-over row, one-arm row, lying row, pullover, chin-up, pullup, shrug

Abs: Any Pilates movement, any crunching movement, plank variations, yoga boat pose, bicycles

3·2·1 FOOD LISTS

In the following pages, you'll find suggested snacks and treats that correspond to every 3-2-1 phase and calorie plan. Remember, with the 3-2-1 Weight Loss Plan, you get to eat every 4 to 5 hours. You can have a snack in the morning, another snack in the afternoon or early evening, and a treat if you need one. (You may omit the treat on days you do not crave it and instead enjoy one additional serving of high-quality starch, a serving of fruit, or an additional 2 ounces of lean meat. See page 135 for tips on how to make these swaps.)

You can eat your snacks and treats at any time of day, fitting them in at times that work best for you. The only rule you must follow: You must eat your snacks and treats in the right portions.

The meal plans in Phase 1 and Phase 2 suggest different-size snacks for different calorie levels. In the following pages, you'll find a list of 100-calorie snacks. Use this list to choose morning and afternoon snacks for the 1,200-calorie menus and morning snacks for the 1,500-calorie menus. You'll also find a 150-calorie list. Use it to choose afternoon snacks for the 1,500-calorie menus and morning snacks for the 1,800-calorie menu. Finally, you'll find a 200-calorie snack list. Use it to choose afternoon snacks for the 1,800-calorie menus.

You'll also find two Treat Lists. It's important to remember that the treat portions do not change with the phases—only the variety is different. The Phase 1 Treat List is short and includes healthful treats. The Phase 2 Treat List is extensive and includes just about all treats you can name.

TREAT LISTS

All treats in the following lists contain 100 to 150 calories. Feel free to meander beyond the lists once you reach Phase 2. Just read labels and make sure your treat doesn't total more than 150 calories.

Phase 1 Treat List

When choosing packaged treats, read labels to be sure the brand you buy contains only 100 to 150 calories per serving.

1 medium banana, sliced, with 2 tablespoons light chocolate syrup for dipping

15 strawberries (or 1 cup mixed berries) with 2 generous tablespoons reduced-fat whipped topping

1 baked apple with 1 teaspoon sugar and cinnamon

1 cup natural unsweetened applesauce

10 baked corn tortilla chips with 2 to 4 tablespoons salsa

1 ounce whole wheat pretzels

½ cup low-fat or fat-free pudding, any flavor

1 low-fat ice cream pop

1 frozen 100% fruit juice bar

½ cup low-fat ice cream, frozen yogurt, or sorbet

1 small bag soy crisps

1 ounce vegetable chips

4 cups light popcorn

2 graham crackers (4 squares), plain or cinnamon

1 ounce dark chocolate

1 serving low-fat hot cocoa with 1 graham cracker (2 squares)

6 ounces red or white wine

12 ounces light beer

1.5 ounces vodka, gin, or tequila

Phase 2 Treat List

When choosing packaged treats, read labels to be sure the brand you choose contains only 100 to 150 calories per serving. I've included soft drinks here, but I urge, urge, urge you *not* to waste your treat calories on soda. Use them for foods that provide you with more sustenance and satisfaction.

Cheese Treats

2 ounces feta cheese

2 ounces light Velveeta cheese

2 ounces (4 tablespoons) fat-free cream cheese

1 ounce goat cheese

1 ounce Brie or other soft cheese

1 ounce Swiss cheese

1 ounce Gorgonzola cheese

1 ounce Cheddar cheese

1 ounce Colby/Monterey Jack marbled cheese

1 ounce American cheese

1 ounce part-skim mozzarella cheese

¼ cup crumbled bleu cheese (not packed)

8 cubes small mild Cheddar/Colby cheese

4 slices fat-free cheese

2 Kraft American cheese singles

2 sticks part-skim string cheese (60–70 calories each)

2 tablespoons Cheez Whiz

Salty/Crunchy Treats

100-calorie snack pack (Nabisco Chips Ahoy!, Pepperidge Farm Goldfish, Frito-Lay Doritos, Keebler Right Bites, etc.)

2 ounces fat-free potato chips (30–40 chips)

1 ounce baked potato chips (about 11 chips)

1 ounce SunChips (11 chips)

1 ounce pretzels

2 cups cheese popcorn

2 cups oil-popped salted popcorn

⅔ cup traditional Chex mix

½ cup Cracker Jack

55 Pepperidge Farm Goldfish crackers

16 Wheat Thins

10 saltines

9 Ritz crackers

7 Triscuits

Salty/Crunchy Treats—*continued*

1 ounce Doritos or Tostitos

4 cups light butter microwave popcorn

3 cups Smartfood reduced-fat white Cheddar popcorn

2 cups Boston Light popcorn

4 plain rice cakes

4 melba toasts

2 honey graham crackers (4 squares)

3 tablespoons almonds, cashews, or peanuts

Starchy Treats

½ medium bagel

1 slice French or Italian bread

1 slice raisin bread

1 dinner roll

3 medium plain or sesame breadsticks

1 small piece cornbread

½ large soft pretzel

1 English muffin

1 slice frozen French toast

1 frozen waffle

2 Eggo Nutri-Grain frozen waffles

2 Kellogg's Special K frozen waffles

10 frozen French fries

Candy

26 pieces candy corn

10 small gummy bears

6 pieces Jolly Rancher hard candy

6 pieces butterscotch candy

5 Tootsie Rolls

4 Bit-O-Honeys

3 or 4 caramels

3 Twizzlers

2 Tootsie Pops

1 ounce peanut brittle

1 ounce toffee

1 ounce taffy

Chocolate

1 ounce fudge

1 ounce dark chocolate–covered
  cherries (2 cherries)

1 ounce truffles

1 Reese's peanut butter cup

10 Whoppers malted milk balls

10 Goobers chocolate-covered peanuts

5 chocolate kisses

1 fun-size piece or package (KitKat,
  M&Ms, Peanut M&Ms, 5th Avenue,
  Almond Joy, Milky Way, Snickers, 3
  Musketeers, 100 Grand, Baby Ruth,
  Butterfinger, and other brands with
  150 calories or less)

3 Hershey's miniatures (milk chocolate,
  milk chocolate with peanuts, Krackel,
  Special Dark, Mr. Goodbar)

Desserts/Cookies/Cakes

½ cup pudding or mousse, any flavor

1 or 2 cookies, any brand
  (150 calories or less)

1 small (2" square) brownie

1 ounce pound cake
  (about ⅒ cake)

1 Weight Watchers Smart Ones
  New York–style cheesecake

1 Weight Watchers Smart Ones
  chocolate éclair

10 animal crackers

8 Nilla wafers

4 or 5 small gingersnaps

1 Little Debbie angel food cake

1 Hostess Twinkie

½ doughnut, any type

Frozen Treats

1 Dairy Queen small vanilla
  or chocolate soft-serve
  wafer cone

1 McDonald's small vanilla
  reduced-fat ice cream cone

1 cup Italian ice

1 Skinny Cow/Silhouette ice cream
  cone, any flavor

1 Healthy Choice ice cream sandwich
  or bar, any flavor

1 Klondike Slim-a-Bear ice cream
  sandwich or bar

Frozen Treats—*continued*

½ cup low-fat ice cream, frozen yogurt, sorbet, or sherbet

1 Creamsicle

1 Fudgsicle

1 Good Humor ice cream sandwich

1 Skinny Cow/Silhouette ice cream sandwich or bar, any flavor

1 Breyers Double Churn 100-calorie ice cream cup

1 no-sugar-added Eskimo Pie, any flavor

1 frozen 100% fruit juice bar

1 Weight Watchers ice cream sandwich, bar, or cone

Soft Drinks

12 ounces soda

12 ounces ginger ale

12 ounces sweetened iced tea

8 ounces lemonade or fruit punch, prepared from mix, frozen, or bottled

20 ounces Gatorade

16 ounces Powerade

Coffee/Tea Treats

10 ounces café latte, made with any type of milk

10 ounces Dunkin' Donuts plain or vanilla Latte Lite

10 ounces Dunkin' Donuts Cappuccino, made with any type of milk

10 ounces Dunkin' Donuts flavored tea or coffee, any flavor, made with any type of milk

12, 16, or 20 ounces Starbucks Caffé Americano

12 or 16 ounces Starbucks Cappuccino, made with any type of milk

12 ounces Starbucks Frappuccino light blended coffee, any flavor, no whipped cream

12, 16, or 24 ounces Starbucks Iced Caffé Americano

12, 16, or 24 ounces Starbucks Tazo iced green tea

6.5-ounce can Starbucks Doubleshot coffee drink

Coffee/Tea Treats—*continued*

12 or 16 ounces Starbucks Caffé Mistro/café au lait, made with any type of milk

9.5-ounce bottle Starbucks Mocha Lite Frappucino coffee drink

Alcohol Treats

12 ounces beer, light or regular

6 ounces champagne

6 ounces red, white, or rosé wine

3 ounces dessert wine

1 ounce coffee liqueur

1 ounce crème de menthe

1 ounce Kahlúa

1 jigger (1.5 ounces) gin, vodka, rum, or whiskey

4 ounces (½ can) tequila sunrise

4 ounces (½ can) whiskey sour

SNACK LISTS

Use the following snack lists for Phases 1 and 2. Make sure you choose a snack from a list that corresponds to the meal plan you are using.

100-Calorie Snacks

Dairy Snacks

1 serving strawberry yogurt freeze (page 187)

6 ounces fat-free flavored yogurt

1 cup fat-free milk

½ cup 1% reduced-fat cottage cheese (mixed with optional cinnamon)

1 part-skim string cheese stick

½ medium banana, sliced, with 2 tablespoons fat-free sour cream

1 slice reduced-calorie, whole wheat bread (45 calories or less), toasted and topped with sliced tomato and ¾ ounce reduced-fat cheese

Fruit Snacks

20 whole strawberries

2 plums

1 cup grapes, pineapple chunks, melon cubes, cherries, or berries

1 pear

1 apple

1 large orange

1 large peach

1 small banana, sliced and frozen

½ mango or papaya

½ cantaloupe

1 cup natural unsweetened applesauce

1 whole grapefruit

Nut Snacks

10 almonds or cashews

8 toasted pecans

Peanut Butter Snacks

1 level tablespoon peanut butter or reduced-fat cream cheese with celery

1 level teaspoon peanut butter with 70-calorie mini whole wheat pita bread

Egg Snacks

4 hard-boiled egg whites

1 hard-boiled egg

Hummus/Guacamole/Salsa Snacks

2 tablespoons hummus or guacamole (page 184) with 1 cup raw vegetables

2 heaping tablespoons salsa or low-calorie salad dressing with 1 cup baby carrots (about 16)

Popcorn Snack

3 cups air-popped popcorn (3 tablespoons unpopped)

Soy Snack

½ cup boiled soybeans in the pod, lightly salted

Coffee Snacks

12 ounces skim cappuccino

12 ounces skim café au lait

12 ounces iced skim café latte

150-Calorie Snacks

Dairy Snacks

6 ounces plain or flavored fat-free yogurt with 1 orange (or 2 tablespoons raisins or ¾ cup berries)

6 ounces plain or flavored fat-free yogurt with 2 tablespoons wheat germ

1 medium banana, sliced and mixed with 2 tablespoons fat-free sour cream

1 part-skim string cheese stick with 1 orange (or 1 peach, 1 plum, 1 small apple, or 1 cup grapes)

½ cup fat-free or 1% reduced-fat cottage cheese with ¼ cantaloupe (or ½ banana, ½ mango, ½ papaya, or ¾ cup berries)

½ cup fat-free or 1% reduced-fat cottage cheese with 1 cup baby carrots

1 slice whole grain toast with 1 ounce fat-free or reduced-fat cheese

Fruit Snacks

1 mango or papaya

1 cup canned fruit salad in light syrup

1 to 1½ cups fresh fruit salad (any combination of fruit)

1½ servings of any fruit listed in 100-calorie snacks

Nut Snacks

15 cashews or almonds

12 toasted pecans

¼ cup pistachio nuts in the shell

Peanut Butter Snacks

2 level teaspoons peanut butter with 2 rice cakes (or 70-calorie whole wheat pita bread)

1 level tablespoon peanut butter with ½ sliced apple

Egg Snack

1 hard-boiled egg (or 4 egg whites) with 1 cup baby carrots

Hummus/Guacamole Snack

3 tablespoons hummus or guacamole (page 184) with 1½ cups peppers, celery, or carrots or 2 cups mixed raw broccoli and cauliflower florets

Popcorn Snack

3 cups air-popped popcorn (3 tablespoons unpopped) sprinkled with 2 tablespoons grated Parmesan cheese

Soy Snacks

1 cup boiled soybeans in the pod, lightly salted   150 calories' worth of soy crisps

Granola Bar Snack

1 low-fat granola bar (150 calories or less)

Coffee Snack

12 ounces skim cappuccino, café au lait, or latte with ½ grapefruit (or 1 orange, 1 peach, or ½ banana)

200-Calorie Snacks

Dairy Snacks

6 ounces fat-free flavored yogurt with 2 tablespoons wheat germ and 2 tablespoons raisins or dried cranberries (or ¾ cup berries)

¼ cup fat-free sour cream with 1 medium banana, sliced

1 part-skim string cheese stick with ½ cantaloupe (or 1 apple, 1 pear, or 1 mango)

1 packet instant oatmeal (150 calories or less) made with ½ cup fat-free milk (or make with water and add ½ cup berries or ½ sliced apple and cinnamon)

1 cup fat-free or 1% reduced-fat cottage cheese (mixed with optional cinnamon)

½ cup fat-free or 1% reduced-fat cottage cheese with ½ cup berries and 2 tablespoons wheat germ (or 1 tablespoon chopped walnuts or slivered almonds)

¾ cup fat-free or 1% reduced-fat cottage cheese with 1 cup baby carrots

1 sheet whole wheat matzo with 2 level tablespoons reduced-fat cream cheese and sliced tomato

1 slice whole wheat toast with 1 ounce reduced-fat cheese and sliced tomato

Fruit Snacks

2 cups fresh fruit salad (any combination of fruit)

2 servings of any fruit listed in the 100-calorie snacks

1 apple (or peach or plum) with 10 unsalted almonds or cashews

Nut Snacks

¼ cup almonds, cashews, pecans, soy nuts or peanuts

⅓ cup pistachio nuts or ¼ cup sunflower seeds (each in the shell)

Peanut Butter Snacks

1 level tablespoon peanut butter with 2 rice cakes (or 70-calorie whole wheat pita bread)

1 level tablespoon peanut butter with 1 apple

Egg Snacks

1 hard-boiled egg (or 4 egg whites) with 1 cup fat-free milk

1 hard-boiled egg (or 4 egg whites) with 1 cup baby carrots and 2 tablespoons low-fat dressing

1 hard-boiled egg (or 4 egg whites) with 1 serving of any fruit listed in 100-calorie snacks

Hummus/Guacamole Snack

4 tablespoons hummus or guacamole (page 184) with 2 cups raw vegetables (broccoli florets, cauliflower florets, peppers, celery, or carrots) and one small whole wheat pita

Popcorn Snack

4 cups air-popped popcorn sprinkled with 2 tablespoons grated Parmesan cheese

Soy Snacks

1¼ cups boiled soybeans in the pod, lightly salted

200 calories' worth of soy crisps

Granola Bar Snack

1 low-fat granola bar (200 calories or less)

Coffee Snacks

12 ounces skim cappuccino, café au lait, or latte (80 calories) with 1 serving of any fruit listed in 100-calorie snacks

SELECTED BIBLIOGRAPHY

Chapter 1

Bahr, R., and O. M. Sejersted. "Effect of intensity of exercise on excess postexercise O_2 consumption." *Metabolism* 40(8) (1991): 836–41.

Kaikkonen, H., M. Vrjama, E. Siljander, P. Byman, and R. Laukkanen. "The effect of heart rate controlled low resistance circuit weight training and endurance training on maximal aerobic power in sedentary adults." *Scandinavian Journal of Medicine and Science in Sports* 10(4) (2000): 211–15.

Murphy, E., and R. Schwarzkoph. "Effects of standard set and circuit weight training on excess post-exercise oxygen consumption." *Journal of Applied Sport Science Research* 6(2) (1992): 88–91.

Reynolds, J. "Case study: weight loss: a client finally sees results with a unique circuit training program." *IDEA Health & Fitness Source* (April 2004): 66.

Chapter 2

Bellisle, F., R. McDevitt, and A. M. Prentice. "Meal frequency and energy balance." *British Journal of Nutrition* 77(1 Suppl) (1997): S57–70.

Crovetti, R., et al. "The influence of thermic effect of food on satiety." *European Journal of Clinical Nutrition* 52 (1998): 482–88.

Farshchi, H. R., M. A. Taylor, and I. A. Macdonald. "Decreased thermic effect of food after an irregular compared with a regular meal pattern in healthy lean women." *International Journal of Obesity and Related Metabolic Disorders* 28(5) (2004): 653–60.

Garrow, J. S., M. Durrant, S. Blaza, D. Wilkins, P. Royston, and S. Sunkin. "The effect of meal frequency and protein concentration on the composition of the weight lost by obese subjects." *British Journal of Nutrition* 45(1) (1981): 5–15.

Jenkins, D. J., T. M. Wolever, V. Vuksan, F. Brighenti, S. C. Cunnane, A. V. Rao, A. L. Jenkins, G. Buckley, R. Patten, and W. Singer. "Nibbling versus gorging: metabolic advantages of increased meal frequency." *New England Journal of Medicine* 321(14) (1989): 929–34.

Johnson, C. S., et al. "Post prandial thermogenesis is increased 100 percent on a high-protein, low-fat diet versus a high-carbohydrate, low-fat diet in healthy young women." *Journal of the American College of Nutrition* 21 (2002): 55–61.

Macht, M., and D. Dettmer. "Everyday mood and emotions after eating a chocolate bar or an apple." *Appetite* 46(3) (2006): 332–36. Epub March 20, 2006.

Malik, V. S., M. B. Schulze, and F. B. Hu. "Intake of sugar sweetened beverages and weight gain." *American Journal of Clinical Nutrition* 84(2) (2006): 274–88.

Masheb, R. M., and C. M. Grilo. "Eating patterns and breakfast consumption in obese patients with binge eating disorder." *Behavior Research and Therapy* 44(11) (2006): 1545–53. Epub ahead of print.

Parker, G., I. Parker, and H. Brotchie. "Mood state effects of chocolate." *Journal of Affective Disorders* 92(2–3) (2006): 149–59. Epub March 20, 2006.

Pelkman, C. L., V. K. Fishell, D. H. Maddox, T. A. Pearson, D. T. Mauger, and P. M. Kris-Etherton. "Effects of moderate-fat and low-fat weight loss diets on the serum lipid profile in overweight and obese men and women." *American Journal of Clinical Nutrition* 79(2) (2004): 204–12.

Piers, L. S., K. Z. Walker, R. M. Stoney, M. J. Soares, and K. O'Dea. "The influence of the type of dietary fat on postprandial fat oxidation rates: monounsaturated (olive oil) vs saturated fat (cream)." *International Journal of Obesity and Related Metabolic Disorders* 26(6) (2002): 814–21.

Polivy, J., J. Coleman, and C. P. Herman. "The effect of deprivation on food cravings and eating behavior in restrained and unrestrained eaters." *International Journal of Eating Disorders* 38(4) (2005): 301–9.

Poston, W. S., C. K. Haddock, M. M. Pinkston, P. Pace, N. D. Karakoc, R. S. Reeves, and J. P. Foreyt. "Weight loss with meal replacement and meal replacement plus snacks: a randomized trial." *International Journal of Obesity* (London) 29(9) (2005): 1107–14.

Schulze, M. B., J. E. Manson, D. S. Ludwig, G. A. Colditz, M. J. Stampfer, W. C. Willet, and F. B. Hu. "Sugar-sweetened beverages, weight gain, and incidence of type 2 diabetes in young and middle-aged women." *Journal of the American Medical Association* 292(8) (2004): 927–34.

Segal, K. R., and B. Gutin. "Thermic effects of food and exercise in lean and obese women." *Metabolism* 32(6) (1983): 581–89.

Slavin, J. "Why whole grains are protective: biological mechanisms." *Proceedings of the Nutrition Society* 62(1) (2003): 129–34.

Slavin, J. L. "Dietary fiber and body weight." *Nutrition* 21(3) (2005): 411–18.

St-Onge, M. P., F. Rubiano, W. F. DeNino, A. Jones Jr, D. Greenfield, P. W. Ferguson, S. Akrabawi, and S. B. Heymsfield. "Added thermogenic and satiety effects of a mixed nutrient vs. a sugar-only beverage." *International Journal of Obesity and Related Metabolic Disorders* 28(2) (2004): 248–53.

Suen, V. M., G. A. Silva, A. F. Tannus, M. R. Unamuno, and J. S. Marchini. "Effect of hypocaloric meals with different macronutrient compositions on energy metabolism and lung function in obese women." *Nutrition* 19(9) (2003): 703–7.

Chapter 3

Burleson, M. A. "Effect of weight training exercise and treadmill exercise on post-exercise oxygen consumption." *Medicine & Science in Sports & Exercise* 30(4) (1998): 518–22.

Gillette, C. A., R. C. Bullough, and C. L. Melby. "Post exercise energy expenditure in response to acute aerobic or resistive exercise." *International Journal of Sports Nutrition* 4 (1994): 347–60.

Haltom, R. W. "Circuit weight training and its effects on excess post exercise oxygen consumption." *Medicine & Science in Sports & Exercise* 31(11) (1999): 1613–18.

Murphy, E., and R. Schwarzkoph. "Effects of standard set and circuit weight training on excess post-exercise oxygen consumption." *Journal of Applied Sport Science Research* 6(2) (1992): 88–91.

Short, K., and K. Nair. "The effect of age on protein metabolism." *Current Opinion in Clinical Nutrition and Metabolic Care* 3(1) (2000): 39–44.

Takeshima, N., M. Rogers, M. Islam, T. Yamauchi, E. Watanabe, and A. Okada. "Effect of concurrent aerobic and resistant circuit exercise training on fitness in older adults." *European Journal of Applied Physiology* 93(1-2) (2004): 173–82.

Volpi, E., R. Nazemi, and S. Fujita. "Muscle tissue changes with aging." *Current Opinion in Clinical Nutrition and Metabolic Care* 7(2004): 405–10.

Chapter 4

Baker, R. C., and D. S. Kirschenbaum. "Weight control during the holidays: highly consistent self-monitoring as a potentially useful coping mechanism." *Health Psychology* 17(4) (1998): 367–70.

Boutelle, K. N., and D. S. Kirschenbaum. "Further support for consistent self-monitoring as a vital component of successful weight control." *Obesity Research* 6(3) (1998): 219–24.

Chapter 13

Burke, L. E., S. Sereika, J. Choo, M. Warziski, E. Music, M. Styn, J. Novak, and A. Stone. "Ancillary study to the PREFER trial: a descriptive study of participants' patterns of self-monitoring—rationale, design and preliminary experiences." *Contempory Clinical Trials* 27(1) (2006): 23–33. Epub November 28, 2005.

Carels, R. A., L. A. Darby, S. Rydin, O. M. Douglass, H. M. Cacciapaglia, and W. H. O'Brien. "The relationship between self-monitoring, outcome expectancies, difficulties with eating and exercise, and physical activity and weight loss treatment outcomes." *Annuals of Behavioral Medicine* 30(3) (2005): 182–90.

Elfhag, K., and S. Rossner. "Who succeeds in maintaining weight loss? A conceptual review of factors associated with weight loss maintenance and weight regain." *Obesity Reviews* 6(1) (2005): 67–85.

Gallagher, K. I., J. M. Jakicic, M. A. Napolitano, and B. H. Marcus. "Psychosocial factors related to physical activity and weight loss in overweight women." *Medicine & Science in Sports & Exercise* 38(5) (2006): 971–80.

Green, M. W., N. A. Elliman, and M. J. Kretsch. "Weight loss strategies, stress, and cognitive function: supervised versus unsupervised dieting." *Psychoneuroendocrinology* 30(9) (2005): 908–18.

Harvey-Berino, J., S. Pintauro, P. Buzzell, and E. C. Gold. "Effect of Internet support on the long-term maintenance of weight loss." *Obesity Research* 12(2) (2004): 320–29.

Kristeller, J. L., and C. B. Hallett. "An exploratory study of meditation-based intervention for binge eating disorder." *Journal of Health Psychology* 4(3) (1999): 357–63.

Leigh Gibson, E. "Emotional influences on food choice: Sensory, physiological and psychological pathways." *Physiology & Behavior* 89(1) (2006): 53–61. Epub ahead of print.

Raynor, H. A., and L. H. Epstein. "Effects of sensory stimulation and post-ingestive consequences on satiation." *Physiology & Behavior* 70(5) (2000): 465–70.

INDEX

Underscored page references indicate boxed text and tables. **Boldface** references indicate photographs.

A

Abdominal exercises, 34, 35–36
    body plank, 82, 88–89, **88–89**
    dandasana twist, 57, **57**
    for Phase 3, 312
    Pilates bicycle, 72–73, **72–73**
    reverse curl with toe reach, 81, **81**
    roll back, 64, **64**
Arms circuit, 47
    abs exercises in, 57, **57**
    cardio in, 47–52, **47–52**
    Phase 1, **169–70**
    Phase 2, **259–60**
    strengthening in, 53–56, **53–56**, 312
Artificial sweeteners, 141–42
Avocado
    No-Guilt Guacamole, 184

B

Back circuit, 82
    abs exercises in, 88–89, **88–89**
    cardio in, 82–84, **82–84**
    Phase 1, **173–74**
    Phase 2, **263–64**
    strengthening in, 85–87, **85–87**, 312

Back extension, 82, 87, **87**
Bacon, turkey
    breakfast BLT, 226, 240, 254
    broccoli and mushroom omelet with turkey
        bacon and toast, 232, 246
Balancing biceps curl, 54, **54**
Bananas
    Berry-Banana Smoothie, 269
    Bring-on-the-Morning Smoothie, 180
Bauer, Joy, background of, 8–9
Beans
    black bean and cheese burrito, 221
    black bean and cheese burrito with rice,
        235, 249
    Black Bean Salad, 179
    as protein source, 26
    turkey burger with black bean salad, 148,
        154, 162
    vegetable bean soup with salad, 218, 232,
        246
Bedtime, eating treat before, 19, 20, 136,
    290–91
Beef
    burgers, 130–31
    grilled sirloin, 132

grilled sirloin with mozzarella and tomato salad, 167

grilled sirloin with tomatoes and balsamic dressing, 153, 160

Lean Beef Fajitas, 276

roast beef and brie on a roll, 221, 235, 249

Bend and round, 46, **46**

Berries. *See also* Strawberries

Berry-Banana Smoothie, 269

Bring-on-the-Morning Smoothie, 180

mixed berry and yogurt parfait, 221, 235, 249

old-fashioned oatmeal with berries, 160, 167

waffles with vanilla yogurt and berries, 148, 155, 162

whole grain cereal with berries, 202, 219

whole grain cereal with nuts and berries, 233, 247

Beverages

avoiding extra calories from, 101, 141, 209

for Phases 1 and 2, 141, 146, 209, 215

Biceps curl, 53, **53**

balancing, 54, **54**

Biceps muscle, 47

Bicycle, 65

Pilates, 72–73, **72–73**

Bingeing, 16, 17

Bioelectrical impedance, for measuring body fat, 113

Blood sugar

foods affecting, <u>21</u>, 23, 25

low, 16

BMI. *See* Body mass index

BOD POD, for measuring body fat, 113

Body fat measurements, 112–13

Body mass index (BMI), 108–10, <u>109</u>, 112

Body plank, 82, 88–89, **88–89**

Boredom, preventing eating from, 289

Bowel habits, plateaus from, 111

Breads

broccoli and mushroom omelet with toast, 202, 218

broccoli and mushroom omelet with turkey bacon and toast, 232, 246

English muffin pizza, 225

English muffin pizza with vegetable salad, 239, 253

hard-boiled egg with toasted English muffin and peanut butter, 202, 222, 236, 250

reduced-calorie whole grain, 144

sunny-side-up egg on whole grain toast, 202, 227, 241, 255

toast with cream cheese, tomato, onion, and lox, 217, 231, 245

vanilla-cinnamon French toast, 152, 159, 166

yogurt with peanut butter toast, 151, 158, 165

Breakfast

night eating affecting, <u>14–15</u>, 19

restaurant choices for, 130, 202

in 3-2-1 plan, 18

Broccoli

broccoli and mushroom omelet with toast, 202, 218

broccoli and mushroom omelet with turkey bacon and toast, 232, 246

Whole Wheat Penne with Chicken and Broccoli, 283

Brussels sprouts

grilled wild salmon with brussels sprouts, 149, 156, 163

Buns circuit, 74

abs exercises in, 81, **81**

cardio in, 74–76, **74–76**

Phase 1, **172–73**

Phase 2, **262–63**

strengthening in, 77–80, **77–80**, 312

Burgers

grilled turkey burger with mixed green salad, 204, 229

grilled turkey burger with mixed green salad and baked French fries, 243, 257

Prevention Chicken Burgers, 278

as restaurant meal, 130–31, 204

turkey burger with black bean salad, 148, 154, 162

Burritos

black bean and cheese burrito, 221

black bean and cheese burrito with rice, 235, 249

C

Calcium supplements, 136, 137, 209

Calf stretch, standing, 91, **91**

Calorie burning, sources of, 35, <u>36</u>, <u>37</u>

Calorie control, in 3-2-1 eating plan, 12, 28–29

Calorie counts, analyzing recipes for, 198

Cancer, <u>21</u>, 26, 128

Candle lighting, as end-of-meal ritual, 98

Canned goods, in grocery lists, 144, 212

Carbohydrates. *See also* Starches

high-quality, 20–22

refined, 22, 23, 25, <u>25</u>

Cardio exercise
    benefits of, <u>36</u>
    options for, 311–12
    in 3-2-1 plan, 34 *(see also specific exercises and circuits)*
Carrots
    Sweet Carrots, 188
    turkey-cheese sandwich with baby carrots, 149, 156, 163
Catch a football, 76, **76**
Cauliflower
    Parmesan Pureed Cauliflower, 185
Cereals
    whole grain cereal with berries, 202, 219
    whole grain cereal with milk and fruit, 147, 154, 161
    whole grain cereal with nuts and berries, 233, 247
Cheating, 205, 291–92
Cheese
    black bean and cheese burrito, 221
    black bean and cheese burrito with rice, 235, 249
    Chicken and Spinach Citrus Salad with Feta Cheese, 270
    Eggplant Parmigiana, 272
    grilled sirloin with mozzarella and tomato salad, 167
    judging restaurant portion of, 201
    Mozzarella and Tomato Salad, 183
    omitting, in meal plans, 128
    open-faced grilled cheese and tomato sandwich with vegetable salad, 150, 157, 164
    Parmesan Pureed Cauliflower, 185
    roast beef and brie on a roll, 221, 235, 249
    roasted vegetable and goat cheese sandwich, 227, 241, 255
    turkey-cheese sandwich with baby carrots, 149, 156
Chest circuit, 65
    abs exercises in, 72–73, **72–73**
    cardio in, 65–67, **65–67**
    Phase 1, **171–72**
    Phase 2, **261–62**
    strengthening in, 68–71, **68–71**, 312
Chest fly, 70–71, **70–71**
Chewing gum, 99, <u>99</u>, 288
Chicken
    barbecued grilled chicken with spinach and corn on the cob, 204, 218, 232, 246
    Caesar salad, 131

Caesar salad with grilled shrimp or chicken, 148, 155, 162, 203
chicken and spinach salad, 226
Chicken and Spinach Citrus Salad with Feta Cheese, 270
chicken teriyaki over stir-fried vegetables, 147, 154, 161
Chicken with White Wine and Mushrooms, 181
Crispy Chicken Tenders with Honey-Dijon Sauce, 271
grilled chicken with chickpea salad, 153, 160, 167
Middle Eastern Chicken Salad with Tahini Dressing, 277
Prevention Chicken Burgers, 278
as restaurant meal, 204
Rosemary Chicken with Grilled Zucchini, 279
teriyaki with vegetables, 131
whole wheat pasta primavera with grilled chicken, 219, 233, 247
Whole Wheat Penne with Chicken and Broccoli, 283
Chickpeas
    grilled chicken with chickpea salad, 153, 160, 167
Chili
    Extra-Lean Turkey Chili, 273
Chinese food, steamed, 203, 224, 238, 252
Chutney
    Fresh Mango Chutney, 275
Circuit workouts. *See also specific circuits*
    changing order of, 311
    effectiveness of, 5, 7, 35
    importance of completing, 41
Clothing size and fit, for gauging progress, 111, 285, 286
Condiments
    avoiding extra, in Phases 1 and 2, 141, 209
    in grocery lists, 143, 211
Constipation, <u>27</u>, 285
Cooldown exercises, 90–94, **90–94**
    importance of, 41
    Phase 1, **174–75**
    Phase 2, **264–65**
Corn
    barbecued grilled chicken with spinach and corn on the cob, 204, 218, 232, 246
Cottage cheese
    cantaloupe with cottage cheese and slivered almonds, 202, 224, 238, 252
    cottage cheese with fresh fruit, 131, 152, 159, 166

Cravings
    from low blood sugar, 16
    reducing or preventing, 16–17, 25, 29
Cream cheese
    toast with cream cheese, tomato, onion,
        and lox, 217, 231, 245

D

Dairy products
    in grocery lists, 145, 213
    as protein source, 26
Dandasana twist, 57, **57**
Diabetes, 18, 21, 26
Diets
    bingeing after, 16
    reasons for failure of, 12
Dining out guidelines, 129–32, 201–4
Dinners
    for ending night eating, 20
    Phase 1, 19
        restaurant, 131–32
        vegetables in, 128–29
    Phase 2, 19
        restaurant, 203–4
    preventing overeating of, 101–2
    starches and, 19, 196, 287
Double arm row, 82, 85–86, **85–86**
Dry goods, in grocery lists, 144, 212
Dumbbells, weight of, 40, 310–11

E

Eating plan, 3-2-1
    benefits from, 5, 97
    meal plans in (*see* Phase 1, meal plans;
        Phase 2, meal plans)
    rules of
        following, for weight loss, 29
        100 percent healthy meals and snacks,
            11–12, 20–28
        right number of calories, 12, 28–29
        3 meals, 2 snacks, 1 treat, 11, 12–20
Eggplant
    Eggplant Parmigiana, 272
Eggs
    broccoli and mushroom omelet with toast,
        202, 218
    broccoli and mushroom omelet with turkey
        bacon and toast, 232, 246
    in grocery lists, 145, 213
    hard-boiled egg with toasted English muffin
        and peanut butter, 202, 222, 236, 250
    as protein source, 26
    as restaurant meal, 130, 202

scrambled breakfast wrap, 229, 243, 257
    stuffed western egg-white sandwich, 149,
        156, 163
    sunny-side-up egg on whole grain toast,
        202, 227, 241, 255
    Vegetable Omelet, 191
1,800-calorie plan
    bread in, 144
    calorie breakdowns in, 133, 199
    emergency options for, 133, 198
    fish and shellfish in, 213
    Phase 1, 161–67
    Phase 2, 196, 244–57
    produce in, 214
    spices and sauces in, 211
    staples in, 212
    when to choose, 119, 120, 121
Energy, from carbohydrates, 21
Exercise
    essential types of, 36
    in 3-2-1 plan, 7 (*see also* Fitness routines,
        3-2-1)
        determining calorie level, 120
        for ending plateaus, 287, 292–93
Exercise log, 293, 300

F

Fajitas
    Lean Beef Fajitas, 276
Fat, body, measuring, 112–13
Fats, dietary
    benefits of, 27
    calories in, 27
    reducing, 200
    sources of, 27, 28
    in weight loss diets, 26
    for weight loss maintenance, 303
Fiber, 21, 27, 27
1,500-calorie plan
    bread in, 144
    calorie breakdowns in, 133, 199
    emergency options for, 132, 133,
        198
    fish and shellfish in, 213
    Phase 1, 154–60
    Phase 2, 196, 230–43
    produce in, 214
    spices and sauces in, 211
    staples in, 212
    when to choose, 119, 120, 121
Fish
    avoiding contaminants in, 199
    Baked Fish, 178

Fish *(continued)*
    chilled shrimp cocktail with grilled fish, wild rice, and snow peas, 242, 256
    Fish Kebabs, 274
    garden tuna wrap, 220, 234, 248
    grilled, 131–32
    grilled fish with wild rice and snow peas, 203–4, 228
    grilled wild salmon with brussels sprouts, 149, 156, 163
    in grocery lists, 145, 213
    judging restaurant portion of, 201
    as protein source, 26
    toast with cream cheese, tomato, onion, and lox, 217, 231, 245
    Tuna Salad, 190
    Wild Salmon with Spicy Salsa, 186
Fitness routines
    3-2-1 *(see also specific exercises and circuits)*
        abdominal interval in, 34, 35–36
        benefits of, 4, 34, 35, 97
        choosing, 118–19
        circuits in, 5, 34–35
        heart rate for, 38–39, <u>38</u>, 311
        maximizing results from, 37–41
        Phase 1, 41, 117, 168, **168–75**
        Phase 2, 41, 117, 195, 258, **258–65**
        Phase 3, 41, 309–12
        traditional components of, 33–34
Flavorings, avoiding extra, 141, 209
Flies, 65
    chest fly, 70–71, **70–71**
Fluid retention, plateaus from, 110, 285
Food log, 100–101, 102–3, 286–87, 290, 291, 292, 300
French toast
    vanilla-cinnamon French toast, 152, 159, 166
Front hook, 66, **66**
Front jab, 65, **65**
Frozen dinners, 132–33, 197–98
Frozen foods, in grocery lists, 146, 215
Fruits. *See also specific fruits*
    cottage cheese with fresh fruit, 152, 159, 166
    Fruit 'n Nut Muffins, 182
    in grocery lists, 145, 214
    single servings of, 135
    for weight loss maintenance, 303
    whole grain cereal with milk and fruit, 147, 154, 161

G
Goal setting, for weight loss, 107–10, 286
Grains
    judging restaurant portion of, 201
    whole *(see* Whole grains)
Granola
    melon with yogurt, wheat germ, and low-fat granola, 230, 244
Grocery lists
    Phase 1, 143–46
    Phase 2, 210–15
Grocery shopping, 103
Guacamole
    No-Guilt Guacamole, 184
Gum, chewing, 99, <u>99</u>, 288

H
Hamstring curl, 61, **61**
Hamstring stretch, 94, **94**
Heart disease, <u>21</u>, 26
Heart rate, for fitness routines, 38–39, <u>38</u>, 311
Heart rate monitor, 38, 311
Heel touch, 58, **58**
High blood pressure, 177
Holidays, Phase 2 and, 204–5
Hot dogs
    turkey hot dog with mixed green salad, 219, 233, 247
Hummus
    hummus garden wrap, 223, 237, 251
Hunger
    rating, 100
    reducing or preventing, 6, 25, 29, 200
Hydrogenation, 28
Hypoglycemia, 13, 18

I
Insulin, elevated, 23
Insulin resistance, 18
Iron, in multivitamin, 137

J
Jacks, 59–60, **59–60**
Jog, 48, **48**
Journal writing, for stress reduction, 288
Jump rope, 49–50, **49–50**
Junk food addiction, <u>22–23</u>

K
Knee pushup, 68, **68**
Knee strike, 67, **67**

L

Lactose-free foods, in meal plans, 128, 197
Legs and shoulders circuit, 58
    abs exercises in, 64, **64**
    cardio in, 58–61, **58–61**
    Phase 1, **170–71**
    Phase 2, **260–61**
    strengthening in, 62–63, **62–63**, 312
Lox
    toast with cream cheese, tomato, onion, and lox, 217, 231, 245
Lunch
    for ending night eating, 20
    in 3-2-1 plan, 18
    preventing overeating of, 101–2
    restaurant choices for, 130–31, 203
Lunges, 58
Lunge with shoulder press, 62, **62**

M

Macronutrients, 20. *See also* Carbohydrates; Fat; Protein
Magnesium, in multivitamin, 136
Mambo, 82, **82**
Mangos
    Fresh Mango Chutney, 275
March, 42, **42**, 47, **47**
Meal plans
    calorie levels for (*see also* 1,200-calorie plan; 1,500-calorie plan; 1,800-calorie plan)
    changing, 287
    choosing, 119–23, 198–99
    flexibility with, 6–7
    Phase 1 (*see* Phase 1, meal plans)
    Phase 2 (*see* Phase 2, meal plans)
    reviewing, 103
Meal spacing, 13, 18
Measurements, for gauging progress, 111–12, 285, 286
Meats
    in grocery lists, 145, 213
    judging restaurant portion of, 201
    types to avoid or limit, 26, 128, 197
Melons
    cantaloupe with cottage cheese and slivered almonds, 202, 224, 238, 252
    melon with yogurt, wheat germ, and low-fat granola, 230, 244
    melon with yogurt and wheat germ, 216

Mercury, in fish, 199
Metabolism
    circuit workouts increasing, 7
    factors slowing, 13, <u>37</u>, 108, 121, 286, 301, 310
    regular meals preserving, 13–15
Micronutrients, 20
Mindful eating, 100, 102, 290
Monounsaturated fats, 27
Motivation
    Progress Report and, 142
    strategies for, 5, 7–8, 98–104
    for weight loss maintenance, 299
Muffins
    Fruit 'n Nut Muffins, 182
    Whole-Grain Mini-Muffins, 282
Multivitamin, 136–37, 209
Muscle(s)
    affecting body mass index, 110
    stretching, 41
Muscle gain, plateaus from, 110, 285
Muscle loss, metabolism slowed by, 13, <u>37</u>
Muscle mass, preserving, 15–16, <u>37</u>
Muscle repair, protein for, 25
Mushrooms
    broccoli and mushroom omelet with toast, 202, 218
    broccoli and mushroom omelet with turkey bacon and toast, 232, 246
    Chicken with White Wine and Mushrooms, 181

N

Nibbling, preventing, 289–90
Night eating
    breaking cycle of, 19–20, 290–91
    from low blood sugar, 16
    stories about, <u>14–15</u>, 99
Nutritional information, restaurant, 202
Nuts
    cantaloupe with cottage cheese and slivered almonds, 202, 224, 238, 252
    Fruit 'n Nut Muffins, 182
    as protein source, 26
    whole grain cereal with nuts and berries, 233, 247

O

Oatmeal
    instant oatmeal with soy sausage, 225, 239, 253
    old-fashioned oatmeal with berries, 160, 167

Oatmeal (*continued*)
old-fashioned oatmeal with strawberries, 153
as restaurant meal, 130
Obesity
body mass index indicating, 110
whole grains preventing, <u>21</u>
Oils
in grocery lists, 143, 211
for weight loss maintenance, 303
Omega-3 fatty acids, sources of, 27
Omelets. *See* Eggs
Onions
toast with cream cheese, tomato, onion, and lox, 217, 231, 245
Oranges
chicken and spinach citrus salad, 226
Chicken and Spinach Citrus Salad with Feta Cheese, 270
Overeating
preventing, at meals, 101–2
recovering from, 142, 291–92
from TV watching, 100
Overweight, body mass index indicating, 109–10

P

Pasta
judging restaurant portion of, 201
whole wheat pasta primavera with grilled chicken, 219, 233, 247
Whole Wheat Penne with Chicken and Broccoli, 283
Peanut butter
hard-boiled egg with toasted English muffin and peanut butter, 202, 222, 236, 250
yogurt with peanut butter toast, 151, 158, 165
Peppers
Tomato and Green Pepper Salad, 281
Phase 1
duration of, 5, 117, 127
expected weight loss from, 127
fitness routine, 39–40, 168, **168–75**
meal plans, 127–28
1,800-calorie, 161–67
emergency options for, 132–33
1,500-calorie, 154–60
grocery list for, 143–46
pointers for, 141–42
portions in, 29
recipes for, 177–91

restaurant meals and, 129–32
treats in, 134, 135–36, 195–96, 313, 314
1,200-calorie, 147–53
vegetables in, 128–29
Progress Report, 142
starting, 139
Phase 2
duration of, 5, 117, 195
fitness routine, 39, 40, 195, 258, **258–65**
meal plans
1,800-calorie, 199, 244–57
1,500-calorie, 199, 230–43
grocery list for, 210–15
guidelines for, 196–97, 199, 209–10
portions in, 29
recipes for, 198, 267–83
restaurant meals and, 201–4
splurging and, 304
starches in, 196, 200–201
Treat Lists for, 196, 209, 313, 315–19
1,200-calorie, 199, 216–29
during vacations, holidays, and other challenges, 204–5
Progress Report, 210
Phase 3, 117
duration of, 6
eating strategies, 299–305
fitness routine, 40, 309–12
portions in, 29
Phytochemicals, in carbohydrates, 22
Pilates bicycle, 72–73, **72–73**
Pizza
English muffin pizza, 225
English muffin pizza with vegetable salad, 239, 253
Plateaus, weight loss
causes of, 13, 110–11, 285, 286–87, 288–93
help for, 13, 287
during vacations and holidays, 204–5
Plié squats, 58
Plié squat with shoulder raise, 63, **63**
Pork
broiled pork tenderloin with baked potato and vegetables, 204, 223, 237, 251
Portions
importance of controlling, 28, 29
of Phase 2 starches, 200
restaurant, judging size of, 201
Potatoes
Baked French Fries, 268
broiled pork tenderloin with baked potato and vegetables, 223, 237, 251

grilled turkey burger with mixed green salad and baked French fries, 243, 257

Mexican stuffed baked potato, 229, 243, 257

Poultry. *See also* Chicken; Turkey
in grocery lists, 145, 213
as protein source, 26

Power squat, 83, **83**

Prediabetes, 18

Progress Reports, 142, 210

Protein
benefits of, 15, 16, 25–26
lean, vs. high-fat, 26, 199
in Phase 2, 200
sources of, 25, 26
unlimited, constipation from, 27
for weight loss maintenance, 303

Pumpkin
vanilla-pumpkin breakfast pudding, 223, 237, 251

Pushup(s), 65
advanced, 69, **69**
knee, 68, **68**

Q

Quad stretch, 93, **93**

R

Reach and pull, 45, **45**

Recipes
modifying, 198
Phase 1, 177–91
Phase 2, 267–83

Regular, consistent meals, benefits of, 6, 12–17

Restaurant meals, 6
Phase 1, 129–32
Phase 2, 201–4

Rest breaks, in fitness routine, 39

Reverse curl(s), 74
with toe reach, 81, **81**

Rewards, from weight loss, 104–5

Rice
black bean and cheese burrito with rice, 235, 249
judging restaurant portion of, 201

Rituals, for closing meals, 98–99

Roll back, 64, **64**

Rosemary
Rosemary Chicken with Grilled Zucchini, 279

Runner's stretch, 92, **92**

S

Salad dressings
measuring, 131
Middle Eastern Chicken Salad with Tahini Dressing, 277
for Phase 2, 210
Tahini Dressing, 189

Salads
Black Bean Salad, 179
Caesar salad with grilled shrimp or chicken, 148, 155, 162, 203
chicken and spinach salad, 226
Chicken and Spinach Citrus Salad with Feta Cheese, 270
English muffin pizza with vegetable salad, 239, 253
grilled chicken with chickpea salad, 153, 160, 167
grilled sirloin with mozzarella and tomato salad, 167
grilled turkey burger with mixed green salad, 204, 229
grilled turkey burger with mixed green salad and baked French fries, 243, 257
Middle Eastern Chicken Salad with Tahini Dressing, 277
mixed green salad, 157, 163
Mozzarella and Tomato Salad, 183
open-faced grilled cheese and tomato sandwich with vegetable salad, 150, 157, 164
Tomato and Green Pepper Salad, 281
Tuna Salad, 190
turkey burger with black bean salad, 148, 154, 162
turkey hot dog with mixed green salad, 219, 233, 247
vegetable bean soup with salad, 218, 232, 246

Salmon
grilled, 131–32
grilled wild salmon with brussels sprouts, 149, 156, 162
Wild Salmon with Spicy Salsa, 186

Salsa
Wild Salmon with Spicy Salsa, 186

Salt restriction, 177

Saturated fats, 28

Sausage
instant oatmeal with soy sausage, 225, 239, 253

Scallops
    grilled bay scallops with baked sweet potato
        and vegetables, 240, 254
    grilled bay scallops with vegetables,
        226
Seasonings, for Phases 1 and 2, 142, 209
Setbacks, recovering from, 142, 291–92
Shellfish. *See* Scallops; Shrimp
Shoot a basketball, 75, **75**
Shoulder press
    lunge with, 62, **62**
Shoulder raise(s), 58
    plié squat with, 63, **63**
Shoulders circuit. *See* Legs and shoulders
    circuit
Shoulder stretch, 90, **90**
Shrimp
    Caesar salad with grilled shrimp or
        chicken, 148, 155, 162, 203
    chilled shrimp cocktail with grilled fish,
        wild rice, and snow peas, 242, 256
Sirloin. *See* Beef
Skin fold calipers, for measuring body fat,
    112
Smoothies
    Berry-Banana Smoothie, 269
    Bring-on-the-Morning Smoothie, 180
Snacks
    afternoon, 18–19, 20
    100-calorie, 313, 320–21
    150-calorie, 313, 322–23
    200-calorie, 313, 324–25
    guidelines for, 313
    modifying schedule for, 134
    morning, 18, 20
    pre-portioned, 103
Snow peas
    chilled shrimp cocktail with grilled fish,
        wild rice, and snow peas, 242, 256
    grilled fish with wild rice and snow peas,
        203–4, 228
Soft drinks, giving up, <u>23</u>, <u>24</u>
Soup
    vegetable bean soup with salad, 203, 218,
        232, 246
Soy, as protein source, 26
Soy sausage
    instant oatmeal with soy sausage, 225, 239,
        253
Spices, in grocery lists, 143, 211
Spicy foods, for weight loss, <u>29</u>

Spinach
    barbecued grilled chicken with spinach
        and corn on the cob, 204, 218, 232, 246
    chicken and spinach salad, 226
    Chicken and Spinach Citrus Salad with
        Feta Cheese, 270
    sautéed spinach, 224, 238, 252
Squat(s)
    in buns circuit, 74
    with front kick, 80, **80**
    with knee lift, 79, **79**
    with leg lift, 77–78, **77–78**
    power, 83, **83**
    wide rolling, 43, **43**
Standing calf stretch, 91, **91**
Starches
    allowed in Phase 2, 196, 200–201
        substitutions for, 197
    removing, from dinner, 287
    replacing refined grains with, 199
    single servings of, 135
    for weight loss maintenance, 303
Step hop, 52, **52**
Step touch, 51, **51**
Step touch with a soccer kick, 74, **74**
Strawberries
    old-fashioned oatmeal with strawberries, 153
    Strawberry Yogurt Freeze, 187
Strength training
    benefits of, <u>37</u>
    for Phase 3, 312
    in 3-2-1 plan, 34 *(see also specific exercises and*
        circuits)
Stress, preventing eating from, 288–89
Stretches
    benefits of, <u>37</u>
    best time for, 41
    hamstring, 94, **94**
    quad, 93, **93**
    runner's, 92, **92**
    shoulder, 90, **90**
    standing calf stretch, 91, **91**
Success stories, <u>14–15</u>, <u>22–23</u>, <u>30–31</u>, <u>95</u>,
    <u>104–5</u>, <u>114–15</u>, <u>122–23</u>, <u>138</u>, <u>206–7</u>,
    <u>294–95</u>, <u>306–7</u>
Sugar, limiting, 23, 25
Supplements, 136–37
Support person, for motivation, 103
Sweet potato
    grilled bay scallops with baked sweet potato
        and vegetables, 240, 254

T

Tahini
    Middle Eastern Chicken Salad with Tahini
        Dressing, 277
    Tahini Dressing, 189
Tea drinking, as end-of-meal ritual, 99
Thermic effect of eating, 13–15, 26
3-minute meal, 133, 198
Thyroid gland, metabolism and, 13
Tomatoes
    breakfast BLT, 226, 240, 254
    grilled sirloin with mozzarella and tomato
        salad, 167
    grilled sirloin with tomatoes and balsamic
        dressing, 153, 160
    Mozzarella and Tomato Salad, 183
    open-faced grilled cheese and tomato
        sandwich with vegetable salad, 150,
        157, 164
    toast with cream cheese, tomato, onion,
        and lox, 217, 231, 245
    Tomato and Green Pepper Salad, 281
Tooth brushing, as end-of-meal ritual,
    98–99
Torso twist, 44, **44**
Training zone, determining, 39
Trans fat–free products, 28
Trans fats, sources of, 28
Treat Lists, 17. *See also* Treats
    Phase 1, 195–96, 313, 314
    Phase 2, 196, 209, 313, 315–19
Treats, 4, 6, 12, 16–17, 19, 97. *See also* Treat
    Lists
    guidelines for, 134–36, 313
    larger portions of, <u>304</u>, 305
    for night eaters, 20, 290–91
Triceps dip, 55, **55**
Triceps dip II, 56, **56**
Triceps muscle, 47
Trigger foods, 17, 19
Tuna
    garden tuna wrap, 220, 234, 248
    mercury in, 199
    Tuna Salad, 190
Turkey
    bacon
        breakfast BLT, 226, 240, 254
        broccoli and mushroom omelet with
            turkey bacon and toast, 232, 246
    burgers, 130–31, 204
    Extra-Lean Turkey Chili, 273

    grilled turkey burger with mixed green
        salad, 204, 229
    grilled turkey burger with mixed green
        salad and baked French fries, 243, 257
    open-faced turkey Reuben sandwich, 216,
        230, 244
    sandwich, 131
    turkey burger with black bean salad, 148,
        155, 162
    turkey-cheese sandwich with baby carrots,
        149, 156, 163
    turkey hot dog with mixed green salad, 219,
        233, 247
TV watching, overeating and, 100
1,200-calorie plan
    calorie breakdowns in, 133, 199
    emergency options for, 132, 133, 198
    Phase 1, 147–53
    Phase 2, 196, 216–29
    when to choose, 119, 120, 121

U

Underwater weighing, for measuring body
    fat, 112
Unlimited food lists, pros and cons of, <u>203</u>

V

Vacations, following Phase 2 during, 204–5
Vegetables. *See also specific vegetables*
    broiled pork tenderloin with baked potato
        and vegetables, 223, 237, 251
    chicken teriyaki over stir-fried vegetables,
        147, 154, 161
    grilled bay scallops with baked sweet potato
        and vegetables, 240, 254
    grilled bay scallops with vegetables, 226
    in grocery lists, 145, 214
    in Phase 1 dinners, 128–29
    raw, unlimited, <u>203</u>
    roasted vegetable and goat cheese
        sandwich, 227, 241, 255
    Spicy Vegetable Roll-Ups, 280
    substituting, in Phase 2, 197
    vegetable bean soup with salad, 218, 232, 246
    Vegetable Omelet, 191
    for weight loss maintenance, 303
Vegetarian substitutes, in meal plans, 128, 197
Vitamin A, in multivitamin, 137
Vitamin D3, in calcium supplement, 137
Vitamin K, in multivitamin, 137
V-step, 84, **84**

W

Waffles
  waffles with vanilla yogurt and berries, 148, 155, 162
Warmup exercises, 42–46, **42–46**
  importance of, 41
  Phase 1, **168–69**
  Phase 2, **258–59**
Water drinking, for preventing overeating, 101–2
Weigh-ins, for weight maintenance, <u>300</u>
Weight gain, after reaching goal, 300–301, <u>302</u>
Weight loss
  circuit workouts for, 35
  expected, from 3-2-1 plan, 4, 5, 6, 127
  fat intake and, 26–27
  fiber for, 21
  following 3-2-1 rules for, 29
  metabolism slowed by, 13, 121, 286, 301
  monitoring, 110, 111–13, 285–86
  motivation for (*see* Motivation)
  plateaus in (*see* Plateaus)
  preserving muscle mass during, 15–16
  protein for, 25–26
  rewards from, 104–5
  setting goals for, 107–10, 286
  spicy foods for, <u>29</u>
  3-2-1 plan for
    commitment to, 97
    overview of, 3–8
Weight loss maintenance. *See* Phase 3
Wheat germ
  melon with yogurt, wheat germ, and low-fat granola, 230, 244
  melon with yogurt and wheat germ, 216

Whole grains
  choosing, 200–201
  health benefits from, <u>21</u>
  parts of, 22
  vs. refined grains, 199
Wide rolling squat, 43, **43**
Wild rice
  chilled shrimp cocktail with grilled fish, wild rice, and snow peas, 242, 256
  grilled fish with wild rice and snow peas, 203–4, 228
Wine
  Chicken with White Wine and Mushrooms, 181

Y

Yogurt
  melon with yogurt, wheat germ, and low-fat granola, 230, 244
  melon with yogurt and wheat germ, 216
  mixed berry and yogurt parfait, 221, 235, 249
  Strawberry Yogurt Freeze, 187
  vanilla-pumpkin breakfast pudding, 223, 237, 251
  waffles with vanilla yogurt and berries, 148, 155, 162
  yogurt with peanut butter toast, 151, 158, 165
Yo-yo weight loss and gain, 300–301

Z

Zucchini
  Rosemary Chicken with Grilled Zucchini, 279